Skin
and
Aging Processes

Author

Barbara A. Gilchrest, M.D.

Associate Professor of Dermatology
Tufts University
School of Medicine
Boston, Massachusetts

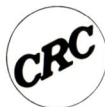

CRC Press, Inc.
Boca Raton, Florida

Library of Congress Cataloging in Publication Data

Gilchrest, Barbara A.
  Skin and aging processes.

  Bibliography: p.
  Includes index.
  1. Geriatric dermatology. 2. Skin--Diseases--Age
factors. 3. Skin--Aging. I. Title.
RL73.A35G54   1984   618.97′6507   83-15051
ISBN 0-8493-5472-2

Direct all inquiries to CRC Press, Inc., 2000 Corporate Blvd., N.W., Boca Raton, Florida, 33431.

© 1984 by CRC Press, Inc.
Second Printing, 1985

International Standard Book Number 0-8493-5472-2

Library of Congress Card Number 83-15051
Printed in the United States

FOREWORD

This is a landmark work. It is the first of its kind which deals comprehensively with cutaneous gerontology. Gilchrest is accomplished both as a clinician and as a researcher, enabling her to achieve a nice blend of both aspects in considerable depth. Thus, one finds terse descriptions of the skin diseases to which the elderly are especially prone intertwined with the findings and theories of diverse investigators who have used the skin as a source material to penetrate the mysteries of the aging process.

Textbooks of gerontology typically pass over the skin lightly or ignore it altogether. Like nearly all physicians, gerontologists are poorly trained in dermatology and find it convenient to avert their eyes from the integument. Besides, people do not die of old skin; it never wears out completely. Also, the skin diseases of the elderly are not death dealing and those few which are, pemphigus, for example, are rare and nowadays even containable, if not curable.

This traditional neglect of the skin is well-nigh unforgivable and has cruel consequences for the well being of the elderly. The great majority of persons over 70 have at least one, often two or three, skin conditions which would benefit from the attentions of a knowledgeable doctor. These disease do not kill but they are persistent pestilences which spoil the quality of life. The elderly themselves expect to have trouble with their skin and do not realize that many of their problems are treatable or preventable.

Gilchrest's thorough exposition of the anatomical and physiologic changes associated with aging provides a sound foundation for understanding the pathogenesis of conditions ranging from xerosis (dry skin) to decubitus ulcers, along with means of combating these.

It is the skin more than any other organ which most clearly reveals the cumulative losses which time prints on the visage of the high and low alike. The cutaneous stigmata of old age — the wrinkles, sags and bags, excrescences, yellowing and mottled pigmentation, leathery roughness — are unsightly and unpleasant. They are also frightening and abhorrent, not only to the ravaged bearer but to all onlookers, especially the calloused young. Gilchrest knows full well the psychological and social costs of this unhandsome, repelling portrait. She is also at pains to use this powerful example to make clear the distinction between intrinsic inevitable aging changes and those which are extrinsic, imposed by ceaseless environmental insults of which sunlight is the major villian. Photoaging is not the same as true aging, and happily is mainly preventable. Time and again we are treated to Gilchrest's insights that various skin diseases are not ineluctable expressions of old age but are rather pathologic processes which are more likely to occur among the elderly, that is, they are age-associated not age-caused.

Because the skin is so large, so regionally diversified, so accessible and manipulable, it is a marvelous tissue for experimental gerontologists. This holds especially for in vitro models of cellular aging. There are elegant technologies to bring into culture the varied cell types. For example, kerainocytes, fibroblasts, melanocytes, Langerhans cells, etc. Moreover, one can easily graft skin for multiple purposes, locally alter it to observe healing, insult it by chemicals or ultraviolet radiation to follow the inflammatory responses, force it to sweat or turn pale or red, endless possibilities for experimental maneuvers which can inform us of the physiologic changes that a young human or animal experiences in the transit to old age.

Finally, no one should suppose that this book has been written solely for dermatologists or medical practitioners. Gilchrest has reviewed a large literature and has forged a systematic synthesis which will make this work useful to different kinds of specialists with an interest in gerontology, viz, cell biologists, anatomists and histologists, physiologists, physicians, and immunologists.

The subject is quite well wrapped up in this volume which will be a handy source work for scientists and doctors who want to know a good deal more than is available in all the dermatologic texts put together.

Albert M. Kligman, M.D., Ph.D.
Philadelphia, PA

INTRODUCTION

Recent decades have witnessed a remarkable increase in our understanding of healthy and diseased skin on the one hand and of the human aging process on the other. The interface of these two fields, cutaneous gerontology and geriatrics, is now emerging as an appropriate focus of attention for medical scientists and clinicians.

The reasons behind this nascent interest in aging skin are complex, but relate in part to demographic considerations: The proportion of elderly citizens in our population has more than tripled in this century. By 2030 more than 20% of Americans will be 65 years or older and 45% of these will be over 75 years old. These individuals require a vastly disproportionate amount of medical care, and in the 1980s the 12% of Americans who are elderly already consume more than half of the federal health budget. The burden of dermatologic disease in the elderly is large and poorly documented. It is psychosocial as well as medical, and although mortality is low, morbidity is high. Furthermore, it is now recognized that illness in the elderly differs qualitatively as well as quantitatively from that in younger adults. Signs and symptoms are often not those listed in standard texts, multiple disorders are the rule rather than the exception, physiologic reserves are decreased, and response to medications may be drastically altered. Little consideration has been given to the impact of cutaneous aging on the presentation of disease or its response to treatment. A major objective of the following chapters is to raise these important issues.

Beyond these clinical considerations lies the potential usefulness of the skin as a model in which to study aging. It is not only the largest and most accessible organ in the body, but contains at least seven well-characterized cell types of varying embryologic origins and differentiated roles. These cells and the cutaneous subunits they compose provide an opportunity to study a wide range of physiologic activities as a function of age both in vivo and in vitro.

Finally, for those of us never formally introduced to gerontology and geriatrics during our professional training, this book may raise new issues of both philosophical and practical importance.

Books are always presumptuous. This is especially true in a poorly defined area for which the audience remains unidentified. The present attempt is best viewed as a nidus for organizing existing knowledge relevant to cutaneous aging and for attracting the interest of today's students, clinicians, and scientists whose task it must be to improve and apply this data base. Dr. Fuller Albright expressed the thought very well in concluding his 1943 Harvey Lecture:

The author is aware that there has been a goodly sprinkling of metaphysics, among this recording of some experimental facts; (s)he is very well aware that the deductions will not all stand the test of time; (s)he does hope, however, that thoughts will be stimulated by this presentation — if not by truths, why then by errors; 'Apologiae' are there none.

I wish to express my gratitude to Dr. Jack Rowe, Head of the Division on Aging, Harvard Medical School, who kindled my own interest in aging; and to Dr. Al Kligman, a creative and productive leader in this field (as in so many others) for the past 30 years, for his generous support of my efforts. Drs. Irwin Braverman, Martin Carter, Bob Goldwyn, Gary Grove, Bob Lavker, Ron Marks, George Martin, Joe McGuire, Donald Murphy, Sheldon Pinnell, Mitch Sams, Ed Schneider, and many others have contributed to this book through their own investigations, interest in and critical analyses of cutaneous aging processes. A very special thanks is owed Ms. Leora Wristen, without whose typing skills the manuscript would never have left my desk.

Barbara A. Gilchrest, M.D.
Boston, MA
March, 1983

THE AUTHOR

Barbara A. Gilchrest, M.D., received her bachelors degree in Mathematics from the Massachusetts Institute of Technology in 1967 and graduated cum laude from the Harvard Medical School in 1971. After 2 years of training in internal medicine on the Harvard Service at Boston City Hospital, she entered the Harvard Dermatology Program, where she completed her clinical training and a 1-year photobiology fellowship. Dr. Gilchrest then spent 1 year as a Research Associate at MIT in Dr. Howard Green's laboratory gaining familiarity with various tissue culture techniques.

In 1977 Dr. Gilchrest joined the Department of Dermatology and Division on Aging faculties at the Beth Israel Hospital and Harvard Medical School. With support from the National Institute on Aging (NIA), Dr. Gilchrest established a tissue culture laboratory to study the effect of habitual sun exposure on the aging process in human skin. Eventually these studies were expanded to include investigation of age-associated loss of proliferative capacity at the cellular level and the development of improved tissue culture systems for keratinocytes and melanocytes derived from human epidermis. During this time Dr. Gilchrest also pursued previous clinical interests in photobiology, phototherapy, and cutaneous aspects of renal failure.

In 1983 Dr. Gilchrest joined the USDA Human Nutrition Research Center on Aging at Tufts University to expand her work on aging and photoaging in skin-derived cells. She also serves as Associate Professor of Dermatology at Tufts University School of Medicine, with comensurate clinical and teaching responsibilities.

Dr. Gilchrest has lectured widely to both professional and lay audiences on aging in the skin, and has developed courses on Geriatric Dermatology for members of the American Academy of Dermatology and on the Biology and Physiology of Aging for Harvard Medical School students. Concerned with increasing physician awareness of age-associated skin problems and with securing adequate federal support for research in gerontologic dermatology, she served as first chairperson on the NIA Liaison Task Force of the American Academy of Dermatology and as consultant to the NIA on several occasions.

Dr. Gilchrest is the author of over 75 scholarly articles, reviews, and textbook chapters and is the recipient of two awards for her work in cutaneous aging. She lives in Brookline, Massachusetts, with her husband and two young sons.

To Byron,
In appreciation of your constant support

Old age is an infectious chronic disease, characterized by the degeneration of the noble elements and by the excessive activity of the phagocytes.

Metchnikoff, 1904

TABLE OF CONTENTS

Chapter 5
Premature Aging Syndromes Affecting the Skin

Chapter 6
Aging and Skin Cancer

Chapter 1

OVERVIEW

I. DEMOGRAPHY OF SKIN DISEASE IN THE ELDERLY

Increasing interest in all aspects of aging can be attributed in part to the shifting population profile in the U.S. A century ago, only 2% of Americans were over 65 years old; in 1900, the figure was 4%, and in 1980, approximately 11%.[1] In 2030 it is estimated that 20% of the population, 50 million Americans, will be over 65 years old.[2] At present, a 65-year-old man has a 13-year life expectancy and a 65-year-old woman has an 18-year life expectancy. From a medical perspective, the 11% of Americans who are elderly occupy one-third of acute care hospital beds[3] and 83% of nursing home and chronic care hospital beds.[4] They account for 30% of the $160 billion spent annually for health care in the U.S. and consume more than 50% of the federal health care budget.[3]

Fewer statistics are available concerning the burden of dermatologic disorders in the elderly. However, a federally sponsored examination of more than 20,000 noninstitutionalized Americans revealed that 40% of those aged 65 to 74 years suffered from a skin disease sufficiently severe in the opinion of the consulting dermatologist to warrant at least one physician visit and the average affected individual had 1.5 such disorders. The costs to society and the individual for diagnosis and management of dermatologic disease are difficult to determine. However, it has been estimated that at least 7% of all physician visits in the U.S. are prompted primarily or exclusively by disorders of the skin.[6] And although hospitalization is infrequently required for dermatologic disease alone, decubitus ulcers, drug rashes, and other cutaneous disorders may greatly complicate and prolong other hospitalizations for the elderly. Published cost estimates for healing an established decubitus ulcer range up to $10,000,[6a] and the estimated total annual cost to American society for venous stasis ulcers alone has been calculated at $655 million.[6b]

In addition to the medical and surgical disorders conventionally included in calculations of disease burden, one must consider the omnipresent ''normal'' changes in aging skin which may have devastating psychological effects and which may predispose the elderly to certain infections and inflammatory diseases. In our youth-oriented society, the visible signs of aging of the skin and its appendages have a measurable negative impact not only on a person's self-image but also on society's perception of him.[7] The more than $10 billion spent annually in this country for cosmetic products,[8] largely in the vain hope of retarding or reversing aging of the skin, is testimony to the horror with which many people regard this process.

II. THE UTILITY OF SKIN FOR STUDIES OF AGING

The skin is an excellent tissue for gerontologic studies. First, it is the largest and most accessible organ system in the body. Biopsy specimens are relatively easy to obtain, and many totally noninvasive procedures yield useful histologic, biochemical, or physiologic data. Second, it contains at least seven cell types of diverse embryologic origin that are potentially amenable to in vivo and in vitro investigation (Table 1). These well-characterized differentiating cell types may be studied individually as a function of age or in the context of integrated tissue responses. Third, it provides a unique opportunity to investigate the influence of environment, in addition to that of genetic factors, on the aging process. This is possible in our culture because certain body surface areas are habitually exposed throughout life while other ''control areas'' are protected by clothing from sunlight, wind, extremes of temperature, and other percutaneous environmental insults.

Table 1
THE SKIN AS A TISSUE SOURCE FOR IN VIVO AND IN VITRO STUDIES OF THE AGING PROCESS

Cutaneous compartment	Cell type	Embryologic origin	Adequacy of culture systems	Present utilization for in vivo and in vitro studies
Epidermis	Keratinocyte	Ectoderm	+ + +	+ +
	Melanocyte	Neural crest	+	+
	Langerhans cell	Bone marrow	0	0
Dermis	Fibroblast	Mesoderm	+ + +	+ + +
	Endothelial cell	Mesoderm	+ +	0
	Mast cell	Bone marrow	+	0
Subcutaneous fat	Adipocyte	Mesoderm	+	0

The skin consists of three distinct compartments,[9] each containing a variety of cells (Figure 1). The following paragraphs briefly describe the structure and function of these compartments and serve as background for Chapters 3 to 8.

The epidermis is composed primarily of keratinocytes (80 to 90% of all epidermal cells) that function in vivo to make the stratum corneum, the major chemical and mechanical barrier of the body. During embryogenesis, subpopulations of keratinocytes invaginate into the dermis and further differentiate to form the epidermal appendages: hair follicles, sebaceous (oil) glands, and eccrine and apocrine (sweat) glands. Epidermal keratinocytes may be further subdivided into a germinative population, normally restricted to the basal layer; and a terminally differentiated population of cells, occupying the suprabasilar layers, that produce structural fibrous proteins (keratins) and later cross-linked envelopes, ultimately destroy their nucleus and other cytoplasmic organelles and finally are shed from the skin surface.[10] The function of the germinative cells is to produce terminally differentiated cells, although the kinetics and controls for this process in vivo are virtually unknown. The terminally differentiated cells produce the stratum corneum through a process in which each cell participates for approximately 1 month in vivo before being shed from the skin surface into the environment. Recent work suggests that basilar keratinocytes may be subdivided into morphologically distinct progenitor cells and other cells that function primarily in dermo-epidermal adhesion.[11]

The second major cell type of the epidermis is the melanocyte, a neural crest derivative that migrates into the fetal epidermis during the 13th week of gestation.[12] Melanocytes constitute approximately 2 to 3% of cells in the epidermis; density varies over the body surface from approximately 1000/mm^2 surface area on the trunk to approximately 2000/mm^2 on the face.[13] The melanocyte is a highly differentiated cell that functions in the epidermis primarily to make melanin pigment granules, protection against damaging solar radiation.[14] The melanocyte is also capable of cell division and migration[15,16] and may influence growth of other cells in the skin.[17]

Langerhans cells are the third major cellular constituent of the epidermis, numbering approximately 300 to 500/mm^2 surface area,[18] 25 to 50% as numerous as melanocytes in most body sites. These cells are bone-marrow derived,[19] possibly transient residents of the epidermis that appear to function primarily in antigen recognition and processing.[20]

The dermis is a complex fibrous matrix set in a mucopolysaccharide gel, through which run blood vessels, lymphatic channels, nerves, glandular ducts, and hair follicles. Cellular constituents of the dermis include fibroblasts, endothelial cells, mast cells, and histiocytes or "fixed tissue macrophages".[9] The fibrous proteins, collagen and elastin, produced by fibroblasts provide tensile strength and elasticity to the skin. The dermal vasculature is the

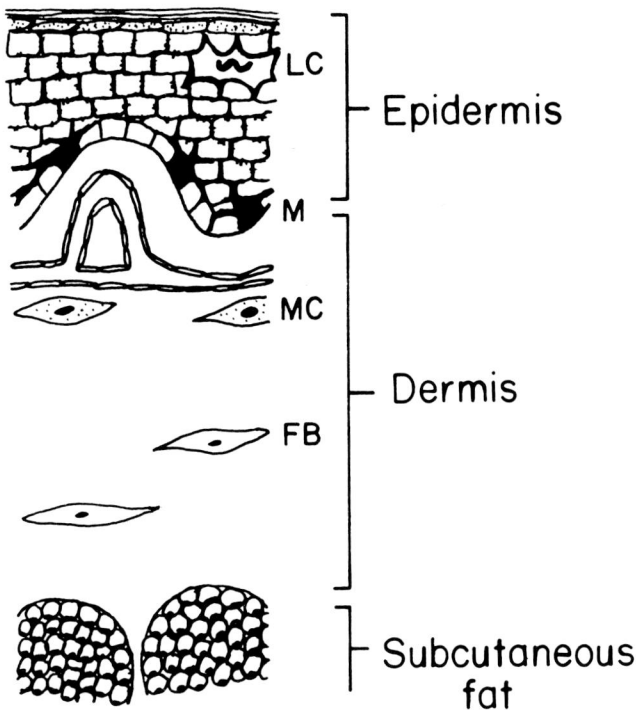

FIGURE 1. Schematic of human skin. The epidermis, dermis, and subcutaneous fat have unique cellular constituents and physiologic functions. The epidermis is entirely cellular, with tightly apposed keratinocytes composing 85 to 90% of the population. These cells continually pass outward in an orderly sequence from the basal layer where mitosis occurs through the progressively differentiated Malpighian layers and granular layer to the stratum corneum, a compact barrier of anucleate squames. Other major epidermal cell types are the melanocyte (M), located in the basal layer, and the Langerhans cell (LC), a migratory cell usually found in the mid-epidermis. The much thicker dermis is composed of extracellular fibrous proteins and mucopolysaccharides; numerous well-organized traversing structures such as capillaries and venules (indicated by a double row of small endothelia cells enclosing a vascular lumen in the superficial dermis); and a variety of cell types including fibroblasts (FB), mast cells (MC), lymphocytes, and histiocytes. In most body locations a layer of subcutaneous fat, composed primarily of adipocytes or "signet cells", separates the dermis from underlying fascia and muscle.

most extensive of any organ system and helps regulate core body temperature through vasoconstriction and vasodilation.

The subcutaneous fat, a layer markedly diminished with age in most body sites, is populated primarily by adipocytes. This layer provides mechanical protection and insulation for underlying structures.

REFERENCES

1. **Besdine, R. W.,** Geriatric medicine, in *Annual Review of Gerontology and Geriatrics,* Eisdorfer, C., Ed,, Springer Publishing Co., New York, 1980, 135.

2. **Kovar, M. G.,** Elderly people: the population 65 years and over, in *Health United States 1976—1977,* National Center for Health Statistics, US DHEW (No. HRS 77-1232), Washington, D.C., 1977.

3. **Gibson, R. M. and Fisher, C. R.,** Age differences in health care spending, fiscal year 1977, *HCFA Health Note,* December, 1978.

4. **Butler, R. N.,** Overview on aging, in *Aging: The Process and the People,* Usding, G. and Hofling, C. J., Eds., Brunner/Mazel, New York, 1978.

5. **Johnson, M. L. T. and Roberts, J.,** Prevalence of dermatological disease among persons 1-74 years of age, United States Advance Data No. 4, US DHEW, Washington, D.C., 1977.

6. **Stern, R. S., Johnson, M. L., and DeLozier, J.,** Utilization of physician services for dermatologic complaints, *Arch. Dermatol.,* 113, 1062, 1977.

6a. **Amberg, R. G., Liggett, I. G., and Wilson, C. G.,** The prevention and treatment of decubitus ulcers in 250 patients, *Orthopedic Review,* 8, 67, 1979.

6b. **Sawyer, P. N., Sophie, Z., Dowbak, G., Cohen, M. D. L., and Feller, I.,** New approaches in the therapy of peripheral vascular ulcer, *Angiology,* 22, 666, 1978.

7. **Lutsky, N. S.,** Attitudes toward old age and elderly persons, in *Annual Review of Gerontology and Geriatrics,* Eisdorfer, C., Ed., Springer Publishing Co., New York, 1980.

8. **Weary, P.E.,** Response to cosmetics: proposal for redefinition, *J Am. Acad. Dermatol.,* 1, 68, 1979.

9. **Breathnach, A. S. and Wolff, K.,** Structure and development of the skin, in *Dermatology in General Medicine,* Fitzpatrick, T. B., Eisen, A. Z., Wolff, K., et al., Eds,, McGraw-Hill, New York, 1979, 41.

10. **Green, H.,** The keratinocyte as differentiated cell type, *Harvey Lect.,* 74, 101, 1979.

11. **Lavker, R. M. and Sun, T. T.,** Heterogeneity in epidermal basal keratinocytes: morphological and functional correlations, *Science,* 215, 1239, 1982.

12. **Rawles, M. E.,** Origin of pigment cells from the neural crest in the mouse embryo, *Physiol. Zool.,* 20, 248, 1947.

13. **Szabo, G.,** Quantitative histological investigations on the melanocyte system of the human epidermis, in *Pigment Cell Biology,* Gordon, M., Ed., Academic Press, New York, 1959, 99.

14. **Thomson, M. L.,** Relative efficiency of pigment and horny layer thickness in protecting the skin of Europeans and Africans against solar ultraviolet radiation, *J. Physiol.,* 127, 236, 1955.

15. **Jimbow, K., Roth, S., Fitzpatrick, T. B., and Szabo, G.,** Mitotic activity in non-neoplastic melanocytes in vivo as determined by histochemical autoradiographic and electron microscopic studies, *J. Cell Biol.,* 66, 663, 1975.

16. **Rosdahl, I. K. and Szabo, G.,** Mitotic activity of epidermal melanocytes in UV-irradiated mouse skin, *J. Invest. Dermatol.,* 70, 143, 1978.

17. **Gilchrest, B. A., Karassik, R., Wilkins, L., and Maciag, T.,** Autocrine and paracrine growth stimulation by normal human keratinocytes, fibroblasts, and melanocytes, *J. Cell. Physiol.,* in press.

18. **Aberer W., Schuler, G., Stingl, G., Honigsmann, H., and Wolff, K.,** Ultraviolet light depletes surface markers of Langerhans cells, *J. Invest. Dermatol.,* 76, 202, 1981.

19. **Katz, S. I., Tamaki, K., and Sachs, D. H.,** Epidermal Langerhans cells are derived from cells which originate in bone marrow, *Nature (London),* 282, 324, 1979.

20. Special issue on dendritic and lymphocytic cells in the epidermis, *J. Invest. Dermatol.,* 75, 1, 1980.

Chapter 2

THE BIOLOGY OF AGING: OBSERVATIONS AND THEORIES

I. INTRODUCTION

The phenomenon of aging is at once obvious and extraordinarily complex. While logic dictates that one or more definable molecular processes within a living organism must underlie the aging process, numerous studies in experimental animals, isolated organ systems, and individual cultured cells and their products have failed to pinpoint the mechanism(s) by which aging occurs. This chapter presents some observations that have excited interest in gerontology and outlines the major hypotheses of aging. More detailed reviews are available in recent texts.[1-4]

II. WHAT IS AGING?

For most people, the term aging evokes an array of clinical findings based on his own experience and his observations of others. In an excellent introductory text,[2] Kohn defines aging in several contexts: (1) chemical aging as manifested by changes in the strucutre of crystals or in macromolecular aggregations; (2) extracellular aging as manifested by progressive cross-linkage of collagen and elastin fibers or by amyloid deposition; (3) intracellular aging as manifested by changes in normal cellular components or by accumulation of substances such as lipofuscin within cells; and (4) aging of entire oganisms. In the general case, aging may be considered an irreversible process which begins or accelerates at maturity and which results in an increasing number and/or range of deviations from the ideal state and/or decreasing rate of return to the ideal state.

Aging is inevitable and every living organism has a finite life span. Moreover, each species has a characteristic maximum attainable life span. Improved nutrition and health care have increased the average human life span from less than 20 years in ancient Greece to over 70 years in the U.S. today, but they have not altered the approximately 110-year maximum life span of our species.[5]

One can consider the phenomenon of maximum life span in another way.[6] If heart disease, currently the leading cause of death in the U.S., were eliminated, the life expectancy at birth would increase only 7 years; and if cancer, the second leading cause of death were eliminated, life expectancy would increase by only 3 years. Indeed, if the 10 leading causes of death were eliminated, life expectancy would increase by less than 11 years. Ultimately, people do not die of pathologic processes but of physiologic processes.

It is interesting that maximum life span, which is so constant within a species, may vary tremendously even among closely related mammals, 86-fold between mice and men, for example.[7] Correlations have been demonstrated between species life span and body weight or brain weight (Figure 1), basal metabolic rate, reproductive rate, and ability to repair DNA damage.[1,8] Although such relationships are provocative, they unfortunately provide little insight into the aging process itself.

III. CHARACTERISTICS OF AGING POPULATIONS

Figure 2 contrasts the survival curves for a population in which death is purely accidental (that is, the risk of death is independent of age and death occurs randomly), and a population in which death is positively related to age and in which there is no accidental death. In Figure 2, the initially trivial or absent death rate begins to increase at a certain age, after

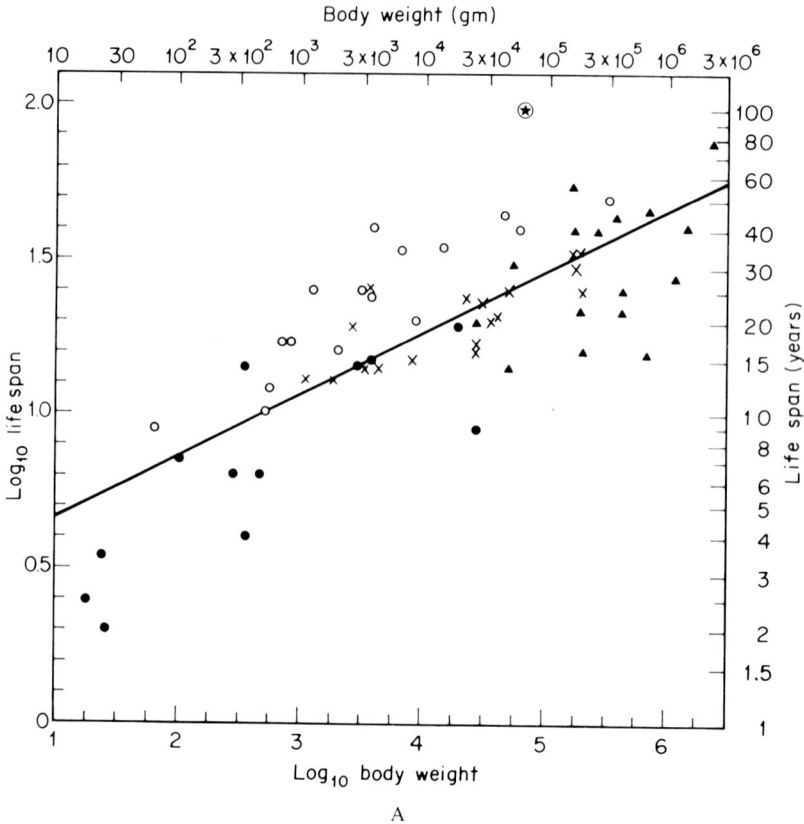

FIGURE 1.   Biologic correlates with maximum species life span. (A) Relationship to body weight. (B) Relationship to brain weight. Sixty-three species of mammals are included in the computations: ○ = primates and lemurs; ● = rodents and insectivores; X = carnivores; ▲ = ungulates and elephants; ⊛ = man. (Reproduced with permission from Sacher G., Relation of lifespan to brain weight and body weight in mammals, in *The Lifespan of Mammals,* Ciba Foundation Colloquiem on Aging, Vol. 5, Little, Brown, Boston, 1959, 115.)

which the percentage of individuals surviving declines rapidly with increasing age. A plot of the death rate in such a population displays a normal distribution. The mathematical relationship of any exponentially increasing death rate with age was articulated more than one and a half centuries ago in what has become known as Gompertz equation:[9] $Q_x = Q_o e^{\alpha x}$, where $Q_x = d_x/hL_x$, the death rate at age x, d_x = the number of deaths between age x and age x + h; L_x = the number alive at age x; Q_o = the initial death rate in the young adult population; and α = a constant for each species. In existing human populations, the distribution is not normal, but reflects a mixture of non-age-related (premature or biologically accidental) deaths, and age-related or senescent deaths (Figure 2).

With improvements in sanitation, nutrition, and medical care, however, the pattern shifts from that of random death to that of Swedish females born in 1961 to 1965 for whom the projection looks almost ideal. Similar progress is evident in the population survival curves for the U.S. during this century. Of the individuals born in 1901, 50% died before age 58 years. For those born in 1948, 50% are predicted to die by age 72 years; and for those born in 1975, the median life span will increase by another 5% to 76 years.

IV. PHYSIOLOGIC CHANGES WITH AGE

Human growth and development are characterized by rapid increases in many functions

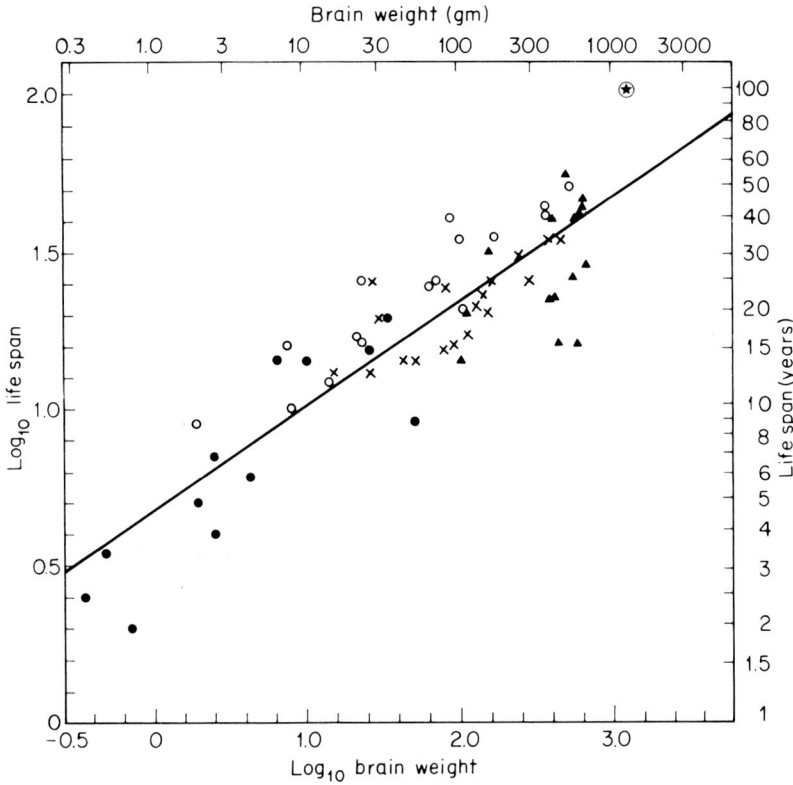

FIGURE 1B

which peak in most cases in early adulthood. Thereafter, virtually all physiologic parameters show a roughly linear decline with age, beginning in the third decade (Figure 3). The changes generally begin immediately at the end of the growth and development phase and generally continue far into old age. There is no pleasant "plateau" during the middle years of peak functional level.

This linearity of functional loss also implies that the *rate* of aging does not increase as we become older. Thus, an 80 year old is aging only as fast as a 30-year-old; he is not losing function at a more rapid rate.

An important characteristic of age-related physiologic changes is their variability. There are several sources of variability, including changes within individuals from organ to organ, and changes from individual to individual in a given population. Variability is present in all populations, but increases dramatically with age.

Some functions such as cardiac output, glomerular filtration rate, and carbohydrate tolerance change rather dramatically, whereas others, such as nerve conduction velocity and hematocrit, undergo no significant change into the eighth or ninth decades. Chapter 3 considers age-associated physiologic decrements in the skin which generally appear to parallel those in other organ systems.

If there is a threshold below which residual physiologic function is incompatible with life, an otherwise healthy aging population would behave as shown in Figure 4. However, such a concept does not explain how the physiologic decrements occur, nor does it predict which functional losses might ultimately be responsible for death.

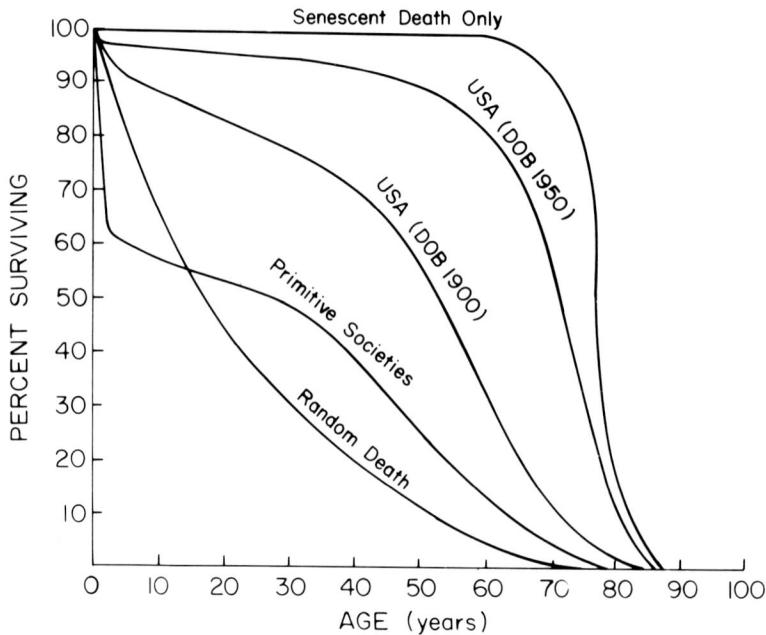

FIGURE 2.   Population survival curves. Idealized curves for populations in which death is truly random and in which death occurs only at the end of a biologically determined 88-year life span are contrasted with actual survival curves for (1) primitive societies with high infant mortality and ''premature'' death rates due to accidents and disease, (2) a moderately advanced society such as the U.S. in the first part of this century (the population cohort born in 1900) and (3) the medically and socially privileged U.S. of the present (the population cohort born in 1950) for whom the curve approaches the ideal of biologically determined senescent death only.

V. AGE VS. DISEASE

Increasing age after adulthood is associated with an exponential increase in mortality rate, and this mortality is preceded by a similar exponential increase in the presence of pathological changes. This has stimulated controversy about whether aging should be considered a disease state, and, if not, what is the relation of normal aging to disease-related changes. There is now general agreement that increasing age is accompanied by inevitable physiologic changes that represent normal aging and are separable from the effects of disease states that become increasingly prevalent with age. These age-related changes are the substrate onto which the effects of specific diseases are grafted. These changes have clinical importance to the physician since they influence the presentation of illness, its response to treatment, and the complications that ensue.

One fairly superficial and simple way of separating disease effects from the influence of normal aging is the inevitability of the changes. Although a change may vary from individual to individual in its age of onset or the rate of loss of function, some loss of function should be demonstrable in all old subjects if the change is due to aging. Aging is a universal phenomenon whereas many disease states, which occur with increasing prevalence as age advances, influence only a small portion of the elderly population. Evaluation of the presence of a change secondary to a disease state or some other factor not age-related in an elderly cohort would often show two populations: one with the effect and one population with no evidence of the effect. The utility of this approach in determining whether or not a change is likely to be related to age can be seen in, as an example, mental failure or senile dementia.

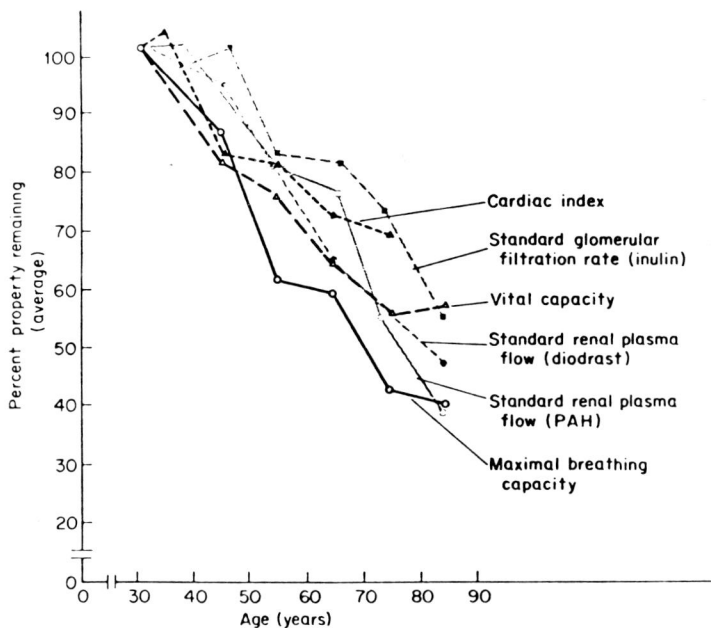

FIGURE 3.   Influence of age on physiologic function in healthy adults. (From Mild-van, A. S. and Strehler, B. L., A critique of theories of mortality, in *The Biology of Aging,* Copyright 1960, by the American Institute of Biological Sciences. Reprinted with permission.)

This loss of mental function with advancing age is thought by some individuals to be characteristic of aging itself. When populations are studied in detail, however, it is shown that dementia occurs in no greater than 10% of elders. Thus, the presence of an intact intellect and the absence of mental failure is consistent with normal aging and is in fact the rule rather than the exception. This would indicate that mental failure cannot be considered a normal consequence of aging but more properly represents a disease that has increasing prevalence in advanced years. This can be contrasted with menopause, which, although variable in its age of onset, is universally present in aged women and thus properly regarded as a result of normal aging.

VI. CELLULAR AGING

A major experimental approach to the mystery of aging has been the study of cultured cells. Alexis Carrel, a surgeon and cell biologist working more than 50 years ago, asked the question: Is an animal's finite life span due to limitations inherent in each individual cell or to mechanisms operative only at the level of the whole organism? Using the relatively primitive tissue culture techniques available at that time, he found chick fibroblasts could be maintained in an actively dividing state for periods far exceeding a chicken's life span[10] and interpreted this to mean individual cells were immortal. As discussed in Chapter 7, these results were later challenged by Hayflick and Moorehead[11] who found that human fetal fibroblasts had a finite, reproducible culture life span after which the cultured cells were incapable of further division and ultimately died.

Hayflick's "aging under glass" model system, in which progression from early to late passage at the cellular level is considered analogous to aging of an organism, has been challenged in turn on the grounds that differences between cells from young and old donors are quantitatively and even qualitatively different from those between early and late passage

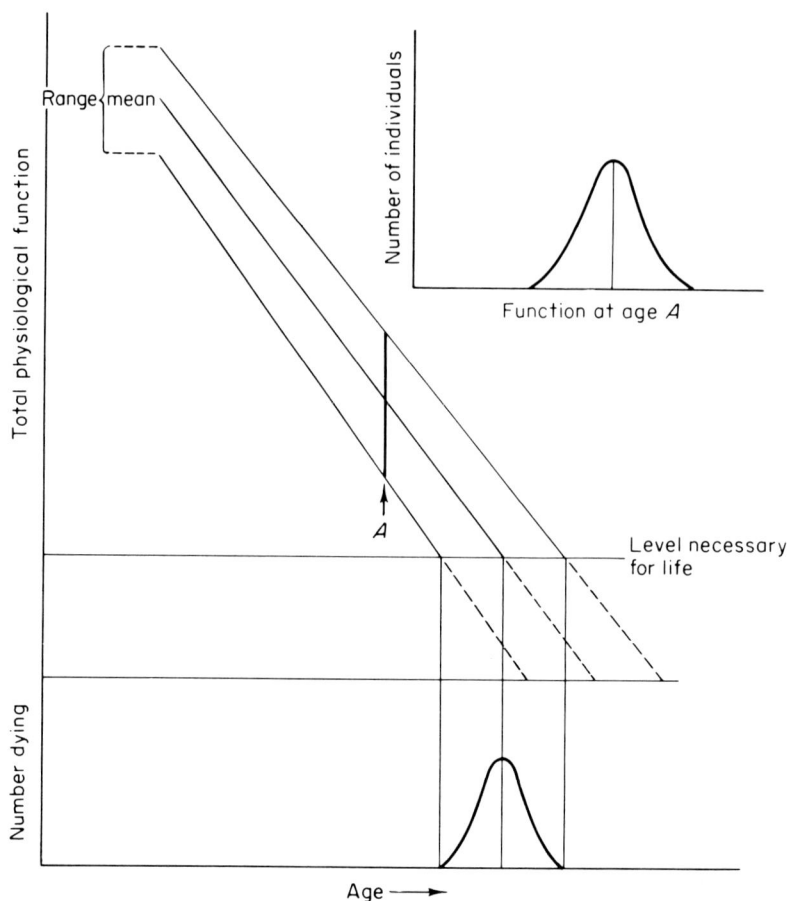

FIGURE 4. Theoretic relationship between physiologic decline and distribution of deaths in an aging population. (From Kohn, R. R., *Principles of Mammalian Aging*, 2nd ed., Prentice-Hall, Englewood Cliffs, NJ, 1978, 179. With permission.)

cultured cells, i.e., aging in vivo differs from "aging" in vitro.[12] Furthermore, analysis of mitotic patterns among cultured fibroblasts indicates that while the cells may be capable on an average of 50 generations, or more correctly of 50 cumulative population doublings, at any point in time the population is a mixture of "old" cells that will never divide again and "young" cells that will undergo many more mitoses.[13] Finally, recent experiments have shown that relatively minor changes in a cultured cell's milieu may increase its culture life span several-fold,[14,15] again raising the issue that subtle environmental inadequacies for cultured diploid cells may be responsible for their limited survival.

An alternative explanation for in vitro senescence is progressive loss of stem cells from cultures in which for practical reasons many cells are discarded at each passage.[16] If cell populations in vivo consist of a few immortal stem cells and many terminally differentiated or "committed" cells capable of only a finite number of divisions, as has been recently postulated for epidermal keratinocytes,[17] serial passage in vitro would ultimately select out those cells with limited life spans.

VII. RELATION OF LIFE SPAN OF CELLS IN CULTURE TO LIFE SPAN OF THE ORGANISM

Four lines of evidence suggest that the life span of normal cultured cells is related to the life span of the organism from which they are derived. First, human dermal fibroblasts[18] and keratinocytes[19] of adult origin have much shorter in vitro life spans than those obtained from fetuses or newborns, and when large numbers of subjects are examined, it becomes apparent that donor age and life span of his cultured fibroblasts are inversely related.[20] Second, fibroblasts from individuals with Werner's syndrome, progeria, and even diabetes — diseases that mimic accelerated aging clinically in some regards — have shorter culture life spans than do those from age-matched controls.[20-24] Third, there is at least a rough correlation between the maximum life span of animal species and in vitro life span of their cultured cells.[25,26] Finally, to answer the nagging question that aging of cells in vitro may be an artifact of tissue culture, rather than a necessary characteristic, several investigators have serially transplanted tissue to isogenic younger animals to determine its maximal life span in vivo. Experiments with skin grafts, bone marrow cells, and mammary tissue have shown that such cells can survive for periods considerably longer than the maximum life span of the species but all die eventually.[27-29] These results are thus consistent with those from tissue culture studies indicating limitation of cell life span.

VIII. THEORIES OF AGING

A. DNA Replication Theory

Deoxyribonucleic acid (DNA), the genetic material of all cells, figures prominently in many theories of aging. It is known that random errors occur, albeit with a very low frequency, during DNA replication. The DNA replication theory states that aging results from a gradual accumulation of such errors, with eventual functional and/or reproductive death of individual cells. In support of this hypothesis, Hart and Setlow[30] have found that life span of animal species, including humans, correlated with the ability of cultured fibroblasts to repair damage to DNA induced by UV radiation (Figure 5). The authors reason that while this specific UV repair capacity would not be expected to determine longevity, the ability to correct DNA errors in general would.

Other investigators have reported an inverse correlation between species life span and cytochrome P-448 content of cultured fibroblasts for six mammalian species including man.[30a] Since cytochrome P-448 is responsible for metabolism of polycyclic hydrocarbons such as dimethylbenzanthracene to their mutagenic (DNA-damaging) forms, the authors suggest that enhanced cellular ability to produce mutagens may result in more rapid aging of the organism and, if so, that aging results from progressive DNA damage.

Other experiments utilizing UV as the DNA insult have been performed with paramecia.[31] These unicellular organisms can reproduce asexually by fission and have a "life span" of approximately 180 divisions after fertilization, roughly equivalent to the life span of cultured diploid cells. Sufficient UV irradiation damages the DNA and not surprisingly reduces the number of divisions the organism can undergo. If, however, one allows photoreactivation, a well-characterized DNA repair process dependent on subsequent visible light or longwave UV exposure, the organisms not only regain their normal division potential, but surpass it, increasing their clonal "life span." The author interprets her work to mean that activation of a specific DNA repair system may also heighten the organism's ability to repair non-UV induced DNA damage and thus retard aging.

A variant of the DNA-error-dependent hypothesis of aging suggests that the number of gene copies for certain critical genes determines the life span of a species.[32] It is known that only 2% of a cell's genetic materials are in use at any time and that multiple copies of at least certain genes exist. If the cell can recognize and replace error-containing genes with undamaged copies, no detrimental effects will occur until the cell has exhausted its genetic reserves.

A genetic program for aging, analogous to the genetic program for development, has been repeatedly postulated, but is thus far unsupported by experimental data.

UNSCHEDULED DNA SYNTHESIS IN YOUNG
FIBROBLASTS EXPOSED TO 254 nm

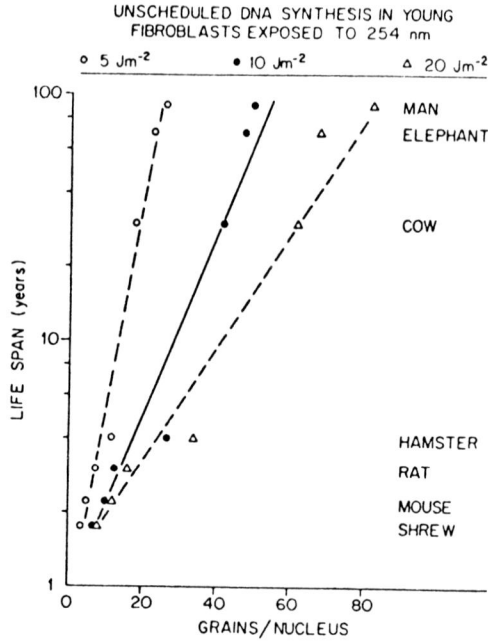

FIGURE 5.   Relationship between DNA repair capacity in UV irradiated cultured fibroblasts and donor species life span. Early passage fibroblast cultures from
seven mammalian species with widely divergent life
spans were exposed to 254 nm radiation in vitro and the
amount of unscheduled DNA synthesis, measured as
grains/nucleus in autoradiographs, was determined after
13 hr, when repair had plateaued. There is good correlation between species life span and level of DNA
repair at all UV fluences examined. (Reproduced from
Hart, R. W. and Setlow, R. B., Correlation between
deoxyribonucleic acid excision-repair and life span in a
number of mammalian species, *Proc. Natl. Acad. Sci.
U.S.A.*, 71(6), 2169, 1974. With permission.)

B. Orgel's Error Theory

Orgel's error catastrophe theory states that even infrequent errors in the transcription of
DNA would produce imperfect RNA molecules, each of which in turn would code for many
faulty enzymes and other proteins. These proteins could accumulate rapidly within the cell
and compromise its function.[33] Progressive loss of functional cells would eventually produce
aging changes and death of the organism.

In support of such a mechanism, most enzyme studies to date have shown an age-dependent
increase in the proportion of partially or totally inactive molecules. In representative cases
a 30 to 70% loss of activity per antigenic unit can be measured between enzymes of young
and old adults.[34] However, several lines of evidence argue against this theory. First, it has
not been possible to detect any change in charge of the altered molecules, even when utilizing
techniques sufficiently sensitive to detect replacement of a single amino acid,[35] while func-
tionally significant transcriptional or translational errors might be expected to replace numerous amino acids. Second, viral infection of early and later passage human fibroblasts
has failed to show a host cell age-dependent increase in production of faulty viral particles.[36]
Third, no correlation was found between in vivo or in vitro age and the rate of mistranslation
in appropriately stressed human fibroblasts; and an immortal, transformed line had a higher

error frequency than did the strains with finite culture life span.[37,38] An alternative explanation for the accumulation with age of functionless proteins without change in charge is post-translational modification.[34] Most amino acid modifications, such as phosphorylation, glycosylation, deamination, and hydroxylation, would again be expected to measurably alter molecular charge or chromatographic properties, but oxidation of sulfhydryl groups, an event already shown to occur in lens protein during cataract formation,[39] would not alter the charge.

C. Cross-Linkage Theory

Bjorkstein[40] and others have hypothesized that aging results from progressive cross-linkage of intracellular and intercellular proteins. Collagen fibers, major structural proteins for many organs that are increasingly cross-linked with age, with a resultant decrease in elasticity and tensile strength, are offered as a prototype. Age-related changes in basement membrane collagen or in the ground substance of connective tissue is postulated to impair organ function. A variant of this theory suggests that progressive covalent bonding of histone protein to DNA is responsible for at least some manifestations of aging.[41]

D. Free Radical Theory

Free radical reactions have been postulated to contribute to biochemical, and ultimately to clinical, aging through progressive membrane damage, protein cross-linkage, enzyme inactivation, and production of "aging pigments".[42] Superoxide and hydroxyl radicals are generated by mitochondrial respiration by autooxidation of numerous intracellular molecules and by the action of certain environmental agents such as UV light on biologic systems. The enzyme, superoxide dismutase, a major cellular defense against damage by free radicals, has been found to decrease as a function of age in rats; and reduced blood levels of other free radical quenchers, including vitamin C, has been reported for elderly human beings. Finally, disputed[41] animal studies suggest that appropriate dietary antioxidants increase the mean life span by 20 to 45% and decrease the incidence of spontaneous carcinoma in genetically predisposed species.[43]

E. "Pacemaker" or Endocrine Theories

Some researchers postulate that aging is controlled by a "pacemaker" such as the thymus, hypothalamus, pituitary, or thyroid gland. Either by elaborating a hormone or by ultimately failing to do so, a single organ might influence the behavior of cells throughout the body. The earliest in vitro aging experiments described an age-associated increase in plasma inhibitor of cellular growth,[10] and one more recent experiment provided evidence for an "aging hormone" of pituitary origin.[44]

F. Immunologic Theory

The immunologic theory of senescence identifies thymus-derived (T) lymphocytes as the pacemaker tissue and states that age-dependent changes in these cells are responsible for much of the pathology that accompanies aging, for example, cancer and certain forms of autoimmunity.[45-47]

REFERENCES

1. **Finch, C. E. and Hayflick, L.,** *Handbook of the Biology of Aging,* Van Nostrand Reinhold Co., New York, 1977, 771.

2. **Kohn, R. R.,** *Principles of Mammalian Aging,* 2nd ed., Prentice-Hall, Englewood Cliffs, N. J., 1978, 240.

3. **Cherkin, A., Finch, C. E., Kharasch, N., Makinoden, T., Scott, F. L., and Strehler, B. L.,** *Aging,* Vol. 8, Physiology and Cell Biology of Aging, Raven Press, New York, 1979, 235.

4. **Rowe, J. W. and Besdine, R. W.,** *Health and Disease in Old Age,* Little, Brown, Boston, 1982, 475.

5. **Shock, N. W.,** *Trends in Gerontology,* 2nd ed., Stanford University Press, Stanford, CA., 1957.

6. **Hayflick, L.,** The cell biology of human aging, *N. Engl. J. Med.,* 295, 1302, 1976.

7. **Denckla, W. D.,** A time to die, *Life Sci.,* 16, 31, 1976.

8. **Sacher, G. A.,** Relation of lifespan to brain weight and body weight in mammals, in *The Lifespan of Animals,* Wolstesholme, G. E. W. and O'Connor, M., Eds., Little, Brown, Boston, 1959, 115.

9. **Gompertz, B.,** On the nature of the function expressive of the law of human mortality and on a new mode of determining life contingencies, *Philos. Trans. R. Soc. London,* 513, 1825.

10. **Carrel, A. and Ebeling, A. H.,** Age and multiplication of fibroblasts, *J. Exp. Med.,* 34, 599, 1921.

11. **Hayflick, L. and Moorehead, P. S.,** the serial cultivation of human diploid cell strains, *Exp. Cell Res.,* 37, 614, 1961.

12. **Schneider, E. L. and Mitsui, Y.,** The relationship between in vitro cellular aging and in vivo human age, *Proc. Natl. Acad. Sci. U.S.A.,* 73, 3584, 1976.

13. **Bell, E., Marek, L. F., Levingstone, D. S., et al.,** Loss of division potential in vitro: aging or differentiation?, *Science,* 202, 1158, 1978.

14. **Rheinwald, J. and Green, H.,** Epidermal growth factor and the multiplication of cultured human epidermal keratinocytes, *Nature (London),* 265, 421, 1977.

15. **Gospodarowicz, D. and Bialeckei, H.,** The effects of the epidermal and fibroblast growth factors on the replicative lifespan of cultured bovine granulosa cells, *Endocrinology,* 103, 854, 1978.

16. **Holliday, R., Huschtscha, L. I., and Kirkwood, T. B. L.,** Cellular aging: further evidence for the commitment theory, *Science,* 213, 1505, 1981.

17. **Lavker, R. M. and Sun, T. T.,** Heterogeneity in epidermal basal keratinocytes: morphological and functional correlations, *Science,* 215, 1239, 1982.

18. **Hayflick, L.,** The limited in vitro lifespan of human diploid cell strains, *Exp. Cell Res,,* 37, 614, 1965.

19. **Rheinwald, J. G. and Green, H.,** Serial cultivation of strains of human epidermal keratinocytes: the formation of keratinizing colonies from single cells, *Cell,* 6, 331, 1975.

20. **Martin, G. I., Sprague, C. A., and Epstein, C. J.,** Replicative lifespan of cultivated human cells. Effects of donor age, tissue, and genotype, *Lab. Invest.,* 23, 66, 1970.

21. **Goldstein, S., Littlefield, J. W., and Soeldner, J. S.,** Diabetes mellitus and aging: diminished plating efficiency of cultured human fibroblasts, *Proc. Natl. Acad. Sci. U.S.A.,* 64, 155, 1969.

22. **Epstein, J., Williams, J. R., and Little, J. B.,** Rate of DNA repair in progeric and normal human fibroblasts, *Biochem. Biophys. Res. Commun.,* 59, 850, 1974,

23. **Goldstein, S.,** Lifespan of cultured cells in progeria, *Lancet,* 1, 424, 1969.

24. **Goldstein, S., Moerman, E. J., Soeldner, J. S., et al.,** Chronologic and physiologic age affect replicative life-span of fibroblasts from diabetic, prediabetic, and normal donors, *Science,* 199, 761, 1978.

25. **Comfort, A.,** *Aging: The Biology of Senescence,* Holt, Rinehart and Winston, Inc., New York 1964.

26. **Hayflick, L.,** The cellular basis for biological aging, in *Handbook of the Biology of Aging,* Finch, C. E. and Hayflick, L., Eds., Van Nostrand Reinhold Co., New York, 1977, 159.

27. **Krohn, P. L.,** Review lectures on senescence. II. Heterochronic transplantation in the study of aging, *Proc. R. Soc. London Ser. B,* 157, 128, 1962.

28. **Daniel C. W., Young, C. J. T., Medina, O., et al.,** The influence of mammogenic hormones on serially transplanted mouse mammary gland, *Exp. Gerontol.,* 6, 95, 1971.

29. **Daniel, C. W.,** Cell longevity: in vivo, in *Handbook of the Biology of Aging,* Finch, C. E., and Hayflick, L., Eds., Van Nostrand Reinhold Co., New York, 1977, 122.

30. **Hart, R. W. and Setlow, R. B.,** Correlation between deoxyribonucleic acid excision-repair and lifespan in a number of mammalian species, *Proc. Natl. Acad. Sci. U.S.A.,* 71, 2169, 1974.

30a. **Pashko, L. L. and Schwartz, A. G.,** Inverse correlation between species life span and specific cytochrome P-448 content of cultured fibroblasts, *J. Gerontol.,* 37, 38, 1982.

31. **Smith-Sonneborn, J.,** DNA repair and longevity assurance in *Paramicium tetraurelia, Science,* 203, 1115, 1979.

32. **Medvedev, Z. A.,** Repetition of molecular-genetic information as a possible factor in evolutionary changes of lifespan, *Exp. Gerontol.,* 1, 227, 1972.

33. **Orgel, L. E.,** The maintenance of the accuracy of protein synthesis in its relevance to aging, *Proc. Natl. Acad. Sci. U.S.A.,* 49, 517, 1963.

34. **Gershon, D., Regnick, A. and Reiss, U.,** Characterization and possible effects of age-associated alterations in enzymes and proteins, in *Aging,* Vol. 8, Physiology and Cell Biology of Aging, Cherkin, A., Finch, C. E., Kharasch, N., Makinoden, T., Scott, F. L., and Strehler, B. L., Eds., Raven Press, New York, 1979, 21.

35. **Gorin, P., Reznick, A. Z., Reiss, U., and Gershon, D.,** Isoelectric properties of nematode aldolase and rat liver superoxide dismutase from young and old animals, *FEBS Lett.,* 84, 83, 1977.

36. **Pitha, J., Stork, E., and Wimmer, E.,** Protein synthesis during aging of human cells in culture, *Exp. Cell Res.,* 94, 310, 1975.

37. **Harley, C. B., Pollard, J. W., Chamberlain, J. W., Stanners, C. P., and Goldstein, S.,** Protein synthetic errors do not increase during aging of cultured human fibroblasts, *Proc. Natl. Acad. Sci. U.S.A.,* 77, 1885, 1980.

38. **Wojtyk, R. L. and Goldstein, S.,** Fidelity of protein synthesis does not decline during aging of cultured human fibroblasts, *J. Cell. Physiol.,* 103, 299, 1980.

39. **Truscott, R. J. W. and Augusteyn, R. C.,** Oxidative changes in human lens protein during senile nuclear cataract formation, *Biochim. Biophys. Acta,* 494, 43, 1977.

40. **Bjorkstein, J.,** The crosslinkage theory of aging, *Finska. Kenists. Medd.,* 80, 23, 1971.

41. **Price, G. B. and Makinodan, T.,** Aging: alteration of DNA-protein information, *Gerontologia,* 19, 58, 1973.

42. **Harman, D.,** The aging process, *Proc. Natl. Acad. Sci. U.S.A.,* 78, 7124, 1981.

43. **Harman, D.,** Prolongation of the normal lifespan and inhibition of spontaneous cancer by antioxidants, *J. Gerontol.,* 16, 247, 1961.

44. **Denckla, W. D.,** Role of the pituitary and thyroid gland in the decline of minimal O_2 consumption with age, *J. Clin. Invest.,* 53, 572, 1974.

45. **Burnet, F. M.,** An immunologic approach to aging, *Lancet,* 1, 353, 1970.

46. **Makinoden, T.,** Immunity and aging, in *Handbook of the Biology of Aging,* Finch, C. E. and Hayflick, L., Eds., Van Nostrand Reinhold Co., New York, 1977, 379.

47. **Kay, M. M. B.,** The thymus: clock for immunologic aging?, *J. Invest. Dermatol.,* 73, 29, 1979.

Chapter 3

AGE-ASSOCIATED CHANGES IN NORMAL SKIN

I. INTRODUCTION

Reflections on the aging process in skin have been offered from time immemorial by both medical and lay authors. Early histologic, physiologic, and biochemical studies of aging human skin are well summarized in the 1964 Symposium on the Biology of the Skin,[1] which clearly portrays the gradual physiologic decline of the organ and increasing individual variability with age.

Recent attempts at organization and critical evaluation of the data base in cutaneous gerontology[2-4] coupled with broader awareness of appropriate strategies for aging research[5] will hopefully permit future investigators to avoid the major pitfalls which complicate interpretations of some earlier work (Figure 1): (1) confusion between aging changes and age-related environmental insults such as chronic sun exposure (e.g., comparison of young and old sun-exposed skin, rather than young and old sun-protected skin); (2) confusion between developmental changes (conception to maturity) and aging changes (maturity to senescence); (3) confusion between aging changes and manifestations of age-associated diseases (e.g., comparison of healthy young adult to debilitated, institutionalized old adults rather than to healthy old adults); and (4) confusion between aging changes and age-associated hormonal changes (e.g., changes in estrogen-responsive skin associated with menopause). Of these, the first is by far the most important, as sun-induced "premature aging" of the skin is widely misunderstood by both physicians and the lay public to be synonymous with the true aging process. In most individuals, sun damage is indeed responsible for the majority of clinically evident age-associated cutaneous changes, but unlike intrinsic aging is readily preventable and relatively well studied.[6] The following sections concern only intrinsic aging unless otherwise specified.

II. MORPHOLOGIC AND HISTOLOGIC CHANGES

The major aging changes in gross morphology of the skin include "dryness" (by which is meant roughness), wrinkling, laxity, uneven pigmentation, and a variety of proliferative lesions.

Histologic features associated with aging in human skin are listed in Table 1. The most striking and consistent change is flattening of the dermo-epidermal junction with effacement of both the dermal papillae and epidermal rete pegs,[7,8] shown schematically in Figure 2. The number of interdigitating papillae and rete pegs per unit skin surface length is also reduced with age, approximately 55% between the third and ninth decades.[9] This results in a considerably smaller contiguous surface between the two compartments[9a] and presumably less "communication" and nutrient transfer, and less resistance to shearing forces.

A. Epidermal Changes

Average epidermal thickness in sun-protected skin probably remains constant with advancing age although deeply invaginated rete pegs are absent. Variability in epidermal thickness and in individual keratinocyte size increases.[10] At the electron microscopic level, sun-protected old skin is characterized by some widening of interkeratinocyte spaces, by reduplication of the lamina densa and anchoring fibril complex in the basement membrane zone; and by loss of the numerous microvillous projections of basal cells into the dermis which greatly increases the dermo-epidermal interface in young adult skin[11] (Figure 3). Similar but more pronounced

Intended for study   Actually studied

                                                Age-associated environmental insults

Intrinsic aging   Development (conception to maturity)
(maturity to
senescence)   Age-associated disease states

                                                Age-associated hormonal changes

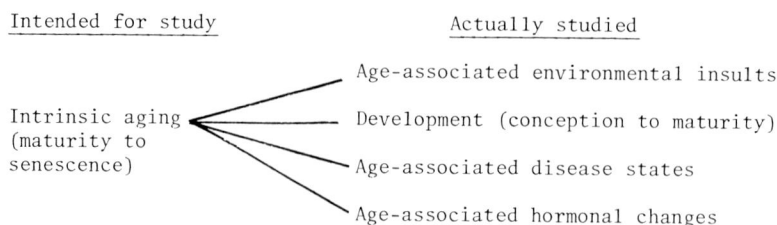

FIGURE 1.   Pitfalls in the study of cutaneous gerontology.

changes in the basement membrane zone are present in old sun-exposed skin.[11] Average thickness and degree of compaction[11] of the stratum corneum appear constant with age. "Skin surface pattern," a patchwork of fine lines which may be determined by papillary dermal architecture, reveal slight age-associated loss of regularity in sun-protected areas, which is much more pronounced in exposed areas.[12]

A decrease in the number of enzymatically active melanocytes per unit surface areas of the skin, approximately 10 to 20% of the remaining cell population each decade, has been repeatedly documented[13-15] (Figure 4). It is not known whether the cells truly disappear or simply become undetectable by ceasing to produce pigment, but in either case the body's protective barrier against UV light is reduced. The number of melanocytic nevi (moles) also progressively decreases with age from a peak of 15 to 40 in the third and fourth decade to an average of 4 per person after age 50, with moles rarely observed in persons beyond age 80.[16]

Bone marrow-derived Langerhans cells, approximately 25 to 50% as numerous as melanocytes, are an epidermal cell population believed to be responsible for recognition of foreign antigens.[17] A nearly 50% reduction in the number of morphologically identifiable epidermal Langerhans cells occurs between early and late adulthood[18] and may account in part for the age-associated decrease in immune responsiveness observed in the skin.

B. Dermal Changes

Loss of dermal thickness approaches 20% in elderly individuals[19,20] (Figure 5) and may account for the paper-thin, sometimes nearly transparent quality of their skin. The remaining dermis is relatively acellular[9] and avascular.[8] Precise histologic concomitants of wrinkling, if any, are unknown, although age-related loss of normal elastin fibers[8] may be contributory.

In one study, an approximately 50% reduction in mast cells and 30% reduction in venular cross-sections were noted in the papillary dermis of buttock skin from old adults compared to young adult controls, and these histologic changes were associated with a corresponding reduction in histamine release and other manifestations of the inflammatory response following a standardized UV light exposure.[21] The consequences of an age-associated loss of dermal mast cells, other than a reduced rate of immediate hypersensitivity reactions such as positive "prick tests"[22] or acute urticaria, are unknown. One study suggests that mast cell-derived heparin plays a role in angiogenesis,[23] a process which may be altered in old skin. In turn, the striking age-associated loss of vascular bed and especially of the vertical capillary loops which occupy dermal papillae in young skin[24] is felt to underlie many of the physiologic alterations in old skin. The marked reduction in the vascular network surrounding hair bulbs, eccrine, apocrine, and sebaceous glands may be responsible for their gradual atrophy and fibrosis with age.

Recent detailed histologic studies of 37 subjects aged 10 to 93 years have stressed the qualitative and quantitative differences between actinic damage and chronologic aging.[25] Forearm skin with mild clinical sun damage revealed marked proliferation of elastic fibers in the papillary dermis; this progressed in severely clinically damaged skin to an increased

Table 1
HISTOLOGIC FEATURES OF AGING HUMAN SKIN

Epidermis	Dermis	Appendages
Flattened dermo-epidermal junction	Atrophy (loss of dermal volume)	Depigmented hair
Variable thickness	Fewer fibroblasts	Loss of hair
Variable cell size and shape	Fewer mast cells	Conversion of terminal to vellus
Occasional nuclear atypia	Fewer blood vessels	hair
Fewer melanocytes	Shortened capillary loops	Abnormal nailplates
Fewer Langerhans cells	Abnormal nerve endings	Fewer glands

number of thickened (up to 20-fold) tangled elastic fibers, and appearance of large elastotic bodies ("solar elastosis"). In contrast, sun-protected buttock skin revealed histologically normal elastic fibers in 9 of 11 subjects aged 18 to 45 years and in 5 of 18 subjects aged 45 to 93 years, with focal loss and/or proliferation of terminal elastic fibers in the remaining subjects. On average, older subjects had thicker elastic fibers (2 to 3 times normal) and fiber alterations deeper in the dermis. Small cysts and lacunae in elastic fibers, first noted in the 30 to 50 year olds, were characteristic of aging sun-protected skin, and progressed to complete fragmentation in many subjects age 70 years. These changes could be experimentally mimicked by incubation of dermal slices with elastase or chymotrypsin (but not collagenase) in vitro suggesting that enzymatic degradation of elastin may be a mechanism for normal dermal aging. The histologic findings were also suggestive of continued synthesis of progressively disorganized elastin throughout adulthood. Increased elastic fibers and histologic evidence of increased elastogenesis were reported in an earlier electron microscopic analysis of aging skin,[11] although differences between sun-exposed and sun-protected skin were felt to be more quantitative than qualitative.

Microvasculature studies in the same histologic sections as the elastic fibers[26] also revealed a divergence between actinic damage and chronologic aging. Capillary and venular walls in sun-exposed skin were thickened by excess basement membrane-like material deposited peripherally, presumably by adjacent veil cells. In contrast, in the nonexposed buttock skin, five of these subjects, aged 59 to 85 years, had normal appearing vessels; three subjects had mild vascular wall thickening; and four subjects, aged 80 to 93 years, had vascular wall thinning to less than half the normal measurement in association with absent or reduced perivascular veil cells (Figure 6). Based on these data, the authors suggest that veil cells are responsible for maintenance of the vessel walls in the dermal microvasculature; that the veil cell is stimulated by repeated sun exposure (or other injuries) to deposit excessive perivascular material; and that with advancing age, the veil cell can no longer meet the demands of normal metabolic turnover in the vessel wall.

C. Appendageal Changes

Age-related changes in hair color, density, and distribution are widely recognized.[27,28] Approximately half the population by age 50 years has at least 50% grey (white) body hair[29] with an even higher proportion of depigmented scalp hair, and virtually everyone has some degree of greying.[30] Greying is due to progressive and eventually total loss of melanocytes from the hair bulb.[13,16] Melanocytes remaining in grey hairs may be vaculated, and the hair matrix and shaft contain fewer melanin granules than normally pigmented hair.[13] Loss of melanocytes is believed to occur more rapidly in hair than in skin because the cells are called upon to proliferate and manufacture melanin at maximal rates during the anagen phase of the hair cycle, while epidermal melanocytes are comparatively inactive throughout their life span. Scalp hair is believed to grey more rapidly than other body hair because its anagen (growth phase) to telogen (resting phase) ratio is considerably greater than that of other body

YOUNG   OLD

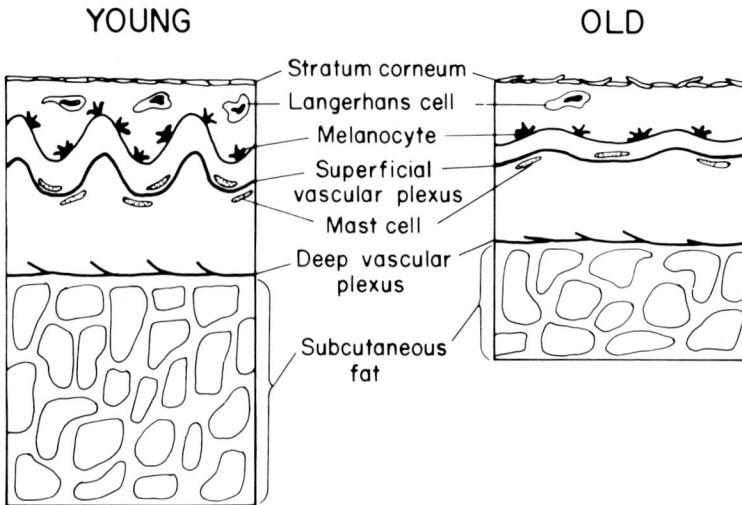

FIGURE 2.   Histologic changes in aging normal skin. Schematic drawings emphasize the age-associated flattening of the dermo-epidermal junction; loss of dermal and subcutaneous mass; shortened capillary loops; and reduced numbers of melanocytes, Langerhans cells, and mast cells. In most body areas, epidermal thickness is approximately 0.1 mm; dermal thickness ranges from 1.0 to 4.0 mm, depending on body site. (From Gilchrest, B., *J. Am. Geriatr. Soc.*, 30, 139, 1982. With permission.)

hair. Advancing age is also accompanied by a gradual decrease in number of hair follicles, from an average density of 615/cm[2] scalp surface in the third decade to less than 500/cm[2] after the fifth decade.[27] Remaining hairs may be smaller in diameter and grow more slowy. The independent process of hair loss on the scalp (balding) results primarily from the androgen-dependent conversion of the relatively dark thick scalp hairs to lightly pigmented short fine hairs similar to those on the ventral forearm.[31]

Bitemporal hair line recession begins during late adolescence in most women and virtually all men.[32] Assessment of baldness is hampered by the difficulty inherent in defining the condition. However, by certain criteria, moderate to advanced bitemporal hair loss among 2650 Englishmen increased in prevalance from 20% at the end of the third decade to more than 60% by the seventh decade, and occipital baldness from less than 3% to more than 25%.[30]

Eccrine glands decrease approximately 15% in average number during adulthood in most body sites,[28] although gland density on the scalp appears constant.[27] Similar quantification has not been performed for apocrine glands. Lipofuscin ("age pigment") gradually accumulates with age in the secretory cells of both eccrine and apocrine glands.[33] Sebaceous gland size and number appear not to change with age,[10] despite evidence of decreased function.

Pacinian and Meissner's corpuscles, the cutaneous end organs responsible for pressure perception and light touch, progressively decrease to approximately one-third their initial average density between the second and ninth decades of life as determined histochemically in two body sites,[34] confirming earlier qualitative observations.[35,36] Further, with advancing age, individuals and organs display greater variation in size and irregularities in structure.[37] There are very few histologically demonstrable aging changes in Merkel's corpuscles or in free nerve endings.[37]

III. PHYSIOLOGIC CHANGES

Table 2 lists the major functions of the skin which decline with age. Many of the entries are necessarily interrelated or overlapping.

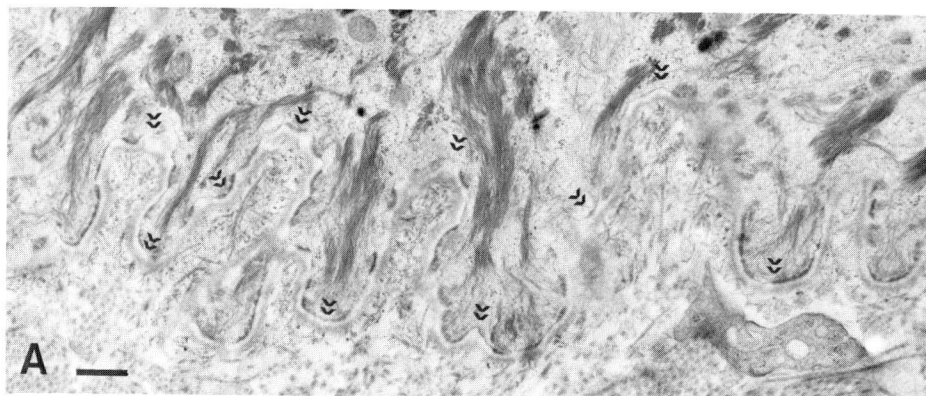

A

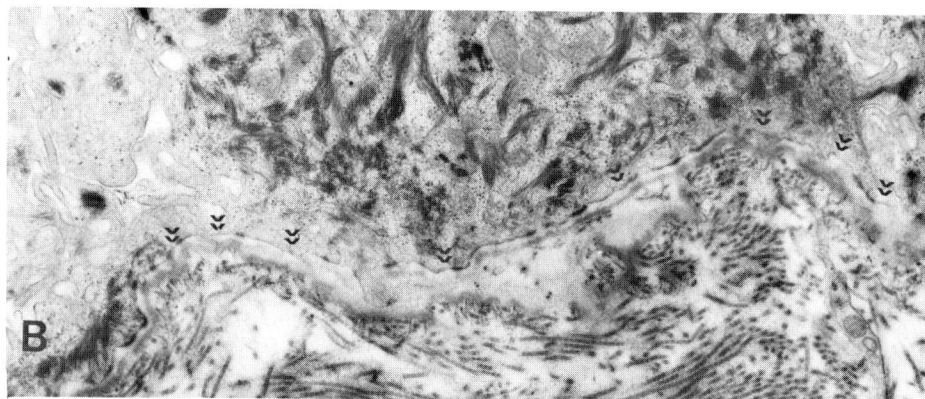

B

FIGURE 3.   Electron micrographs of the dermo-epidermal junction. (A) Upper inner arm of a young adult. Note the numerous microprojections of the basal cell cytoplasma into the papillary dermis. (B) Upper inner arm of an elderly adult. Note absence of basal cell microprojections and resulting decrease in contact surface with the dermis. (Dermo-epidermal junction indicated by double "v" marks. Scale bar = 0.5 μm, photographs × 20,000 (A and B). (Artwork kindly provided by Robert M. Lavker, Ph.D.; modified and reproduced with permission from Lavker, R. M., *J. Invest. Dermatol.*, 73, 59, 1979.)

A. Proliferation and Repair

An age-associated decrease in epidermal turnover rate of approximately 30 to 50% between the third and eighth decades has been determined by a study of desquamation rates for corneocytes (cells of the stratum corneum) at selected body sites[38,39] (Figure 7); similar results in a single study of desquamation rates for scalp corneocytes in patients with dandruff suggest that keratinocyte proliferative capacity decreases with age in diseased as well as normal skin.[38] Thymidine labeling index of the epidermis in vivo has been reported to decline nearly 50% with age, from approximately 5.1% in 19- to 25-year-old men to approximately 2.85% in 69- to 85-year-old men.[24] Other investigators have reported a corresponding 100% prolongation in stratum corneum replacement rate in old vs. young men.[40] Linear growth rates for hair and nails also decrease by approximately 30 to 50% between early and late adulthood.[41]

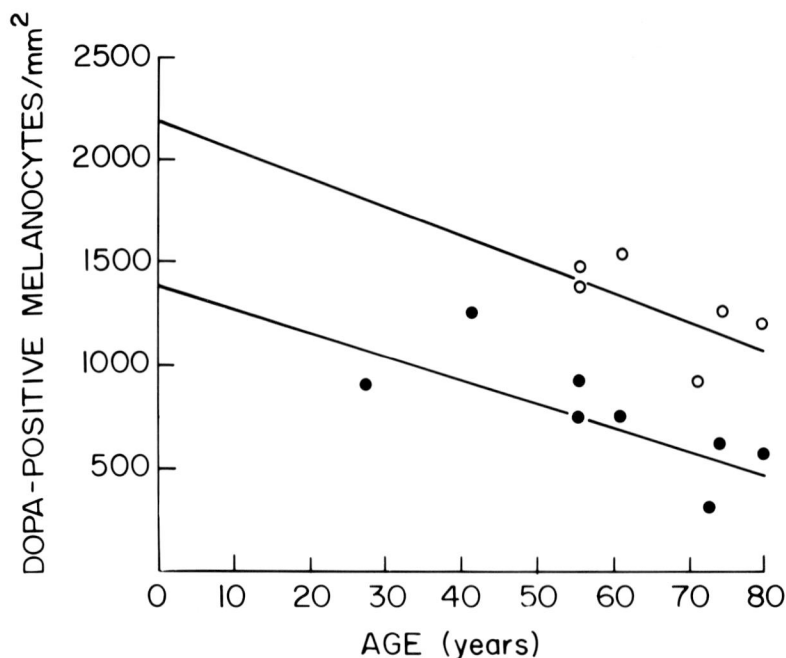

FIGURE 4.   Relationship between age and melanocyte density in habitually sun-exposed skin of the lateral arm (open circles) and nonexposed skin of the medial arm (closed circles) in well-screened fair-skinned adult volunteers without recent sun exposure. Melanocyte counts are the average for 10 independent fields of each split-dopa preparation, viewed at 25 × magnification. The density of dopa-positive cells declines approximately 6 to 8% per decade in both sites, but is consistently higher in habitually (previously) sun-exposed skin. (From Gilchrest, B., et al., *J. Invest. Dermatol.*, 73, 141, 1979. With permission.)

Repair rate in the skin likewise declines with age, whether measured as development of wound tensile strength[42] or collagen deposition,[43] regeneration of excised blister roofs,[44] or excision of thymine dimers in UV-irradiated DNA of cultured dermal fibroblasts.[45] The most extensive of these studies compared the rate of stratum corneum regeneration in 12 subjects aged 18 to 25 years to that in 12 subjects aged 65 to 75 years.[44] Subcorneal blisters were raised by topical application of an ammonium hydroxide solution, the blister roofs excised, and the resulting wound repeatedly observed until normal skin surface markers were restored. This process required a median of approximately 3 weeks in the young subjects but 5 weeks in the old subjects. Healing was essentially complete in all young subjects by 4 weeks; 11 of 12 old subjects were healed by 7 weeks, and the last by 8 weeks.

Neoplasia is associated with aging in virtually all organ systems, but is especially characteristic of skin. One or more of the benign proliferative growths listed in Table 3 is present in nearly every adult beyond age 65 years,[46] and most individuals have dozens of lesions. In the U.S., basal cell carcinoma and squamous cell carcinoma, discussed in Chapter 6, outnumber all other human malignancies combined.[47] These benign and malignant neoplasms almost certainly reflect in part the loss of proliferative homeostasis with age,[48] and perhaps an over-responsiveness to appropriate growth stimuli.

B. Barrier Function and Solute Transfer

Kligman and co-workers have reported an age-related decrease in the barrier function of intact stratum corneum as measured by percutaneous absorption of at least some substances,[49] although the presumably kindred phenomenon of transepidermal water loss did not vary with age for normal adult skin.[24]

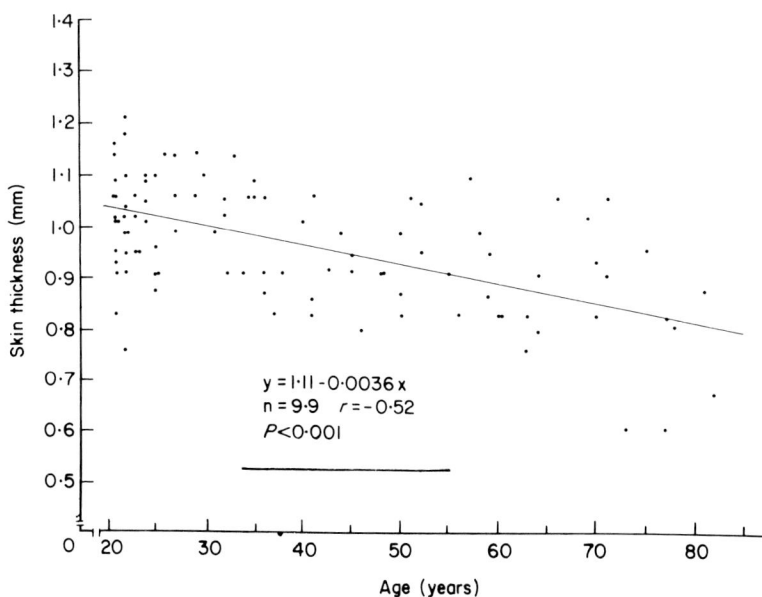

FIGURE 5. Age-associated decrease in skin thickness (epidermis plus dermis). Pulsed ultrasound measurements were made on the flexor aspect of the right mid-forearm of 261 healthy volunteers and plotted as a function of donor age. Values for males (shown in figure) were slightly greater than for females and declined slightly more with age, although statistically significant negative correlations were apparent for both sexes. These in vivo measurements were approximately one-third less than in vitro histiometric measurements of either frozen or formalin fixed biopsies, attributed to artifactual distortion of the processed tissue. (From Tan, C. Y., Statham, B., Marks, R., and Payne, P. A., *Br. J. Dermatol.*, 106, 657, 1982. With permission.)

Aging is also accompanied by a decreased clearance of transepidermally absorbed materials from the dermis,[49] probably due to alterations in the vascular bed and extracellular matrix. Impaired solute transfer between the extravascular and intravascular dermal compartments has been demonstrated in other systems as well, although in some studies it is difficult to isolate the vascular component in a complex inflammatory reaction. After intradermal injection of 0.5 mℓ saline in young and old subjects, resorption from two sun-protected sites required approximately 30 to 65 min in 21 to 30 year olds, but 40 to 110 min in 70 to 83 year olds, with the average time almost twice as long in the elderly[24] (Figure 9).

More recently, the same investigators have also reported the response of young and old adults to topical application of 50% ammonium hydroxide solution (Table 4).[50a] The initial response, characterized by minute perifollicular vesicles, appeared earlier in the old adults and was interpreted by investigators as consistent with either a reduced stratum corneum barrier or an increased shunting of the irritant material through appendageal orifices. Since the average number of horny cell layers, approximately 14 to 17, was identical in the young and old subject groups, decreased barrier function would have to result from a qualitative, not quantitative, change in the stratum corneum. In contrast to the reduced initial response time, however, the time required after vesiculation for development of a tense blister averaged nearly twice as long in the older group, again suggesting a decreased transudation rate with age in injured skin.[50a]

C. Responsiveness to External Stimuli

Decreased sensory perception was documented in old skin more than three decades ago, using several techniques; optimal stimulus in grams for light touch, vibratory sensation, and

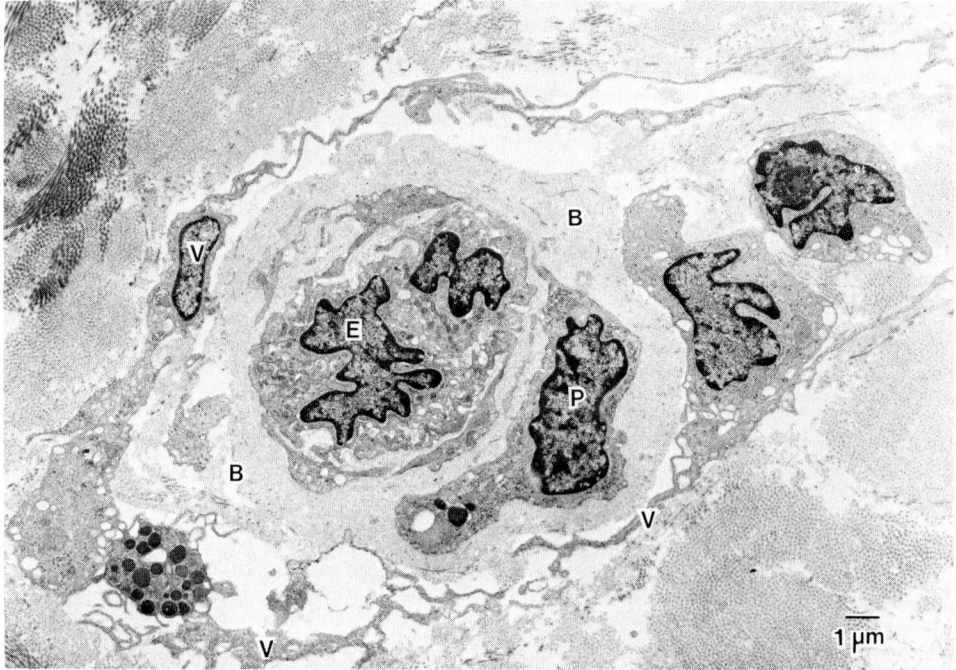

A

FIGURE 6.   Age-associated changes in the cutaneous microvasculature. (A) Mild vascular wall thickening of an arterial capillary, representative of the changes seen in buttock skin biopsies of three of eight older individuals. Veil cells (V) with dilated cisternae are in intimate contact with basement membrane-like material (B) in the vascular wall. Pericyte (P) and endothelial cell (E) appear normal. Vessel wall thickness was within normal limits for the other five older subjects studied and for all six young adult subjects. (B) Abnormally thin wall of a postcapillary venule, representative of the changes seen in buttock skin biopsies of four very elderly (80 to 93 years) subjects. Broad arrowheads indicate sites where vascular wall is reduced to a single basal lamina. Arrows indicate sites where the less dense basement membrane material is markedly decreased, from 2 to 3 μm in young adults to 0.5 to 1 μm. Veil cell (V) appears metabolically inactive, and the number of these cells is reduced. Venous and arterial capillaries were less affected. Similar changes were never seen in young adult subjects. Original magnification ×6457 (A) and ×5904 (B). (Electron micrographs kindly provided by I. M. Braverman, M.D. and reproduced with permission from Braverman, I. M. and Fonferko, E., *J. Invest. Dermatol.*, 78, 444, 1982.)

corneal sensation.[34] Cutaneous pain threshold, defined as reporting discomfort due to quantitated radiant heat focused on a small area of skin, has been reported to increase up to 20% with advancing adult age.[51-54] Unfortunately, the available data do not permit differentiation among several potential explanations for this phenomenon: age-associated increase in the prevalence of peripheral neuropathies[55] (rather than a true aging change in healthy subjects), increased rate of heat dispersion in old skin due to age-associated dermal alterant alterations,[53] an increased peripheral nerve threshold to painful stimuli, or an increased central threshold to pain perception. The clinical significance of these data is further obscured by the many important psychological and social factors influencing an individual's reaction to pain,[56] since all of these may also be presumed to vary with age.

Early studies demonstrated that eccrine sweating is markedly impaired with age. Spontaneous sweating in response to dry heat, measured on digital pads, was reduced more than 70% in healthy old subjects as compared to young control subjects,[57,58] attributable primarily to a decreased output per gland.

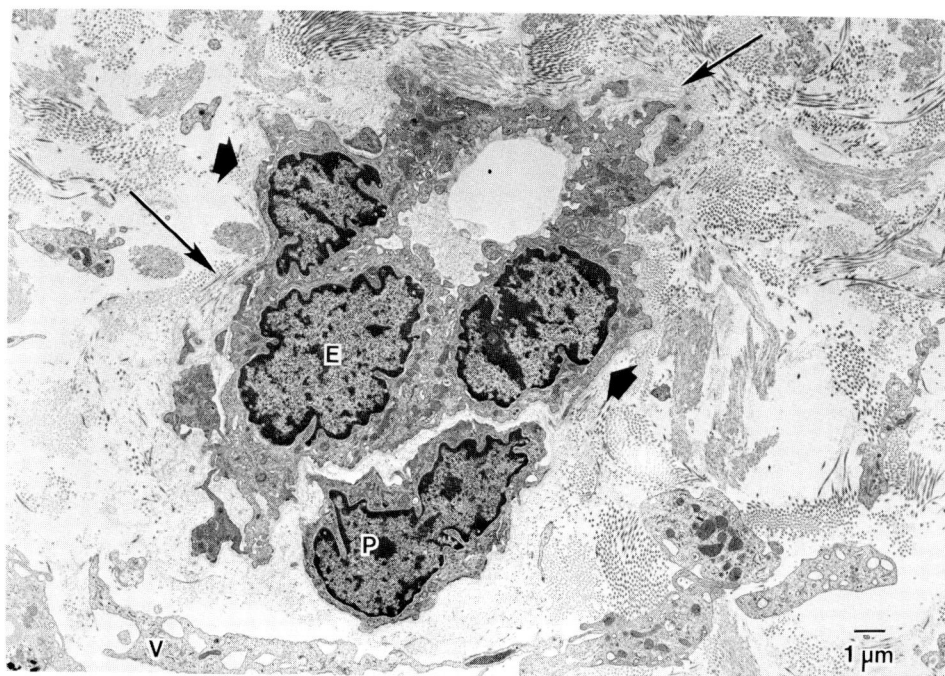

B

Table 2
FUNCTIONS OF HUMAN SKIN
THAT DECLINE WITH AGE

Cell replacement	Immune responsiveness
Injury response	Vascular responsiveness
Barrier function	Thermoregulation
Chemical clearance	Sweat production
Sensory perception	Sebum production
	Vitamin D production

The approximately 60% decrease in sebum production which accompanies advancing age in both men and women is attributed to the concomitant decrease in production of gonadal or adrenal androgen to which sebaceous glands are exquisitely sensitive.[59] The clinical effects of decreased sebum production, if any, are unknown. There is no direct relationship to xerosis or seborrheic dermatitis.

Decreased vascular responsiveness in the skin of older individuals has been documented by clinically assessing vasodilation and transudation after application of other standardized irritants, histamine, and the mast cell degranulating agent 48/80, to young and old skin.[50] Intensity of erythema following a standardized UV exposure is also decreased with age in normal skin,[21] although factors other than decreased vascular responsiveness may be responsible. Compromised thermo-regulation, which predisposes the elderly to hypothermia[60] and possibly heat stroke, may be due in part to reduced vasodilation or vasoconstriction of dermal arterioles, in part to decreased eccrine sweat production, and in part to loss of subcutaneous fat, all of which occur with advancing age.[1]

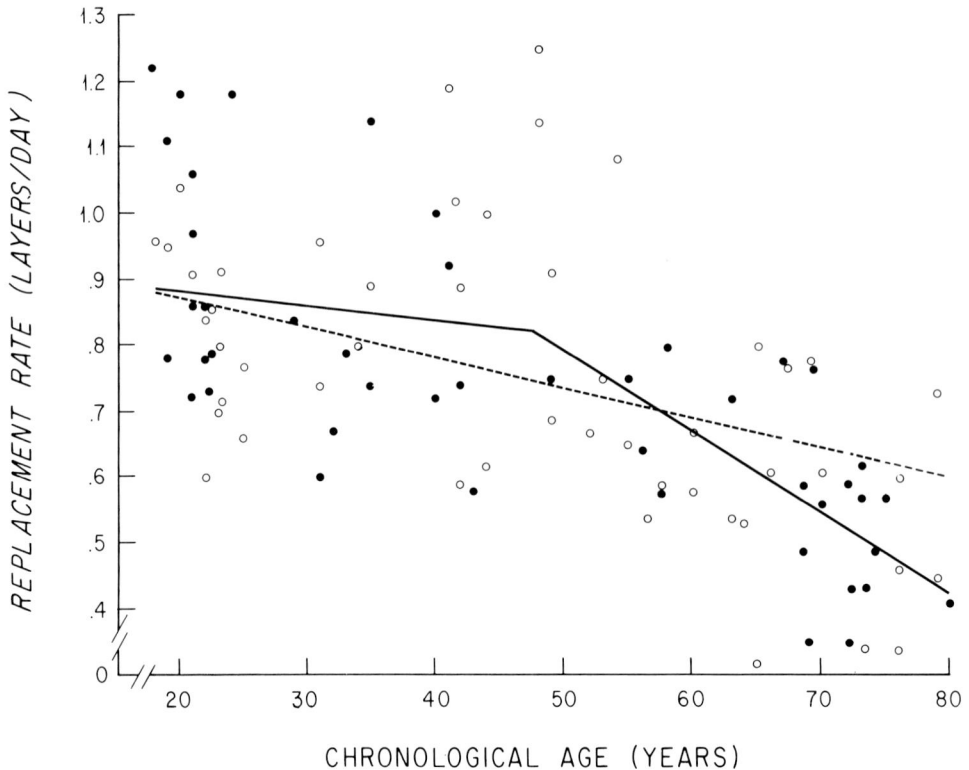

FIGURE 7.   Age-associated decrease in replacement rate for the stratum corneum (SC). Values for healthy adult subjects were calculated by dividing the number of SC cell layers (determined histologically in specially treated excised blister roofs and found not to vary with age) by the SC transit time (determined by disappearance time for a corneocyte-specific dye marker). Best fit regression curves are plotted for both a linear model (---) and a computer-determined hinged linear spline model (——). No differences were apparent between male (●) and female (○) subjects. (From Grove, G. L. and Kligman, A. M., *J. Gerontol.*, 38, 137, 1983. With permission.)

D. Dermo-Epidermal Adhesion

Dermo-epidermal separation has been reported to occur more readily in the elderly under experimental conditions[50,61] (Table 4), as might be anticipated from the histologic finding of reduced interdigitation between the dermis and epidermis.[7,8,11] The poor adhesion between these two cutaneous compartments in the elderly undoubtedly explains their propensity to "torn" skin and superficial abrasions following minor traumas such as bandage removal, and to bulla formation in edematous sites. It may also contribute to the increased prevalence of certain bullous dermatoses in the elderly.[62]

E. Immune Function

An age-associated decrease in delayed hypersensitivity reactions in human skin is manifested by a relative inability of healthy older subjects to develop sensitivity to dinitrochlorobenzene (DNCB) and by their lower rate of positivity for standard test antigens compared to young adult controls. In one study comparing two groups of 45 healthy volunteers, 70% of those younger than 80 years reacted to at least one of five standard recall antigens, whereas only 24% of the octagenarians did.[63] The positivity rates for candidin and trichohytin decreased by twofold and sevenfold, respectively. In another group of 116 healthy subjects, 94% of those below 70 years could be sensitized to DNCB, vs. 69% of those older than 70 years.[64] This decrease undoubtedly reflects the well-documented decrease in total

Wound Healing Following Unroofing of NH₄−OH Blisters On Upper Inner Arms Of Human Subjects

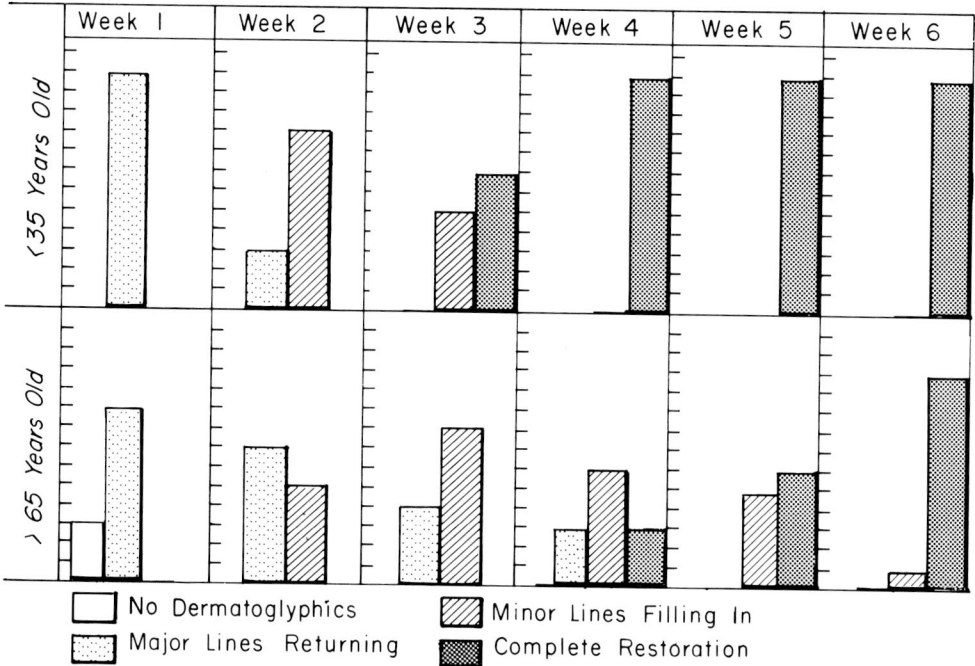

FIGURE 8. Effect of age on superficial wound healing. In two groups of healthy adults, aged 18 to 25 years and 65 to 75 years, blisters were raised on the volar forearm and upper inner arm, the blister deroofed, and the time to healing observed. Healing was more rapid in young than in old subjects, with good correlation between the two sites. (Graphs kindly provided by G. L. Grove, Ph.D. and reproduced in part with permission from Grove, G. L., et al., *J. Soc. Cosmet. Chem.*, 32, 15, 1981.)

Table 3
PROLIFERATIVE GROWTHS ASSOCIATED WITH AGING IN HUMAN SKIN

Lesion	Major participating cells or tissues
Acrochordon (skin tag)	Dermis, keratinocytes, melanocytes
Cherry angioma	Capillaries
Seborrheic keratosis	Dermis, keratinocytes, melanocytes
Lentigo	Melanocytes
Sebaceous hyperplasia	Sebaceous glands

number of circulating thymus-derived lymphocytes and in their responsiveness to standard mitogens,[65] as well as the above-mentioned local cutaneous changes.

The decrease with age in cutaneous manifestations of immediate hypersensitivity is equally pronounced. In one well-controlled epidemiologic study of over 300 subjects in Arizona, the percent with at least one positive wheal-and-flare reaction to a standard battery of potential

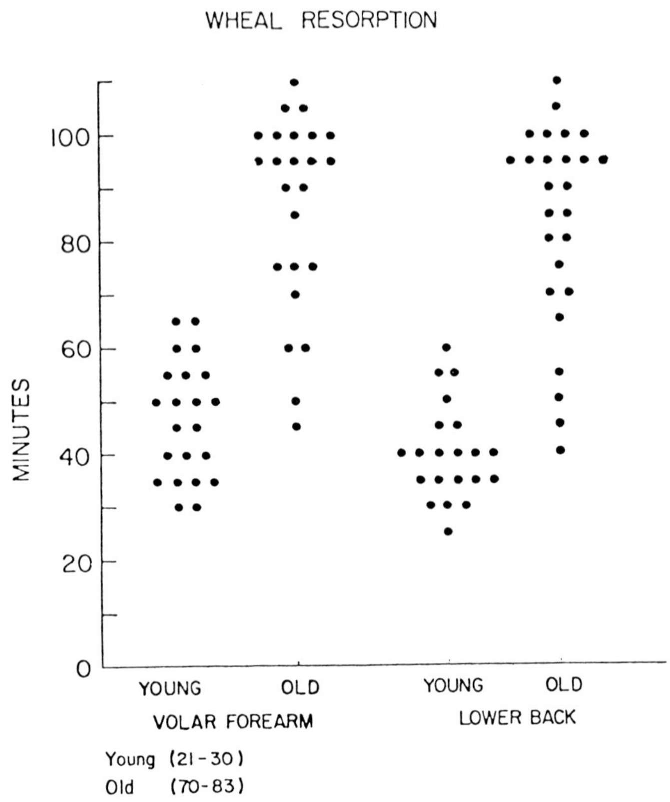

WHEAL RESORPTION

FIGURE 9.   Affect of age on wheal absorption. (From Kligman, A. M., J., *Invest. Dermatol.*, 73, 39, 1979. With permission.)

Table 4
BLISTERING RESPONSES IN RELATION
TO AGE AND SITE

Site	Initial response time (min)	Blister formation time (min)
Volar forearm		
Young adult	11.6 ± 4.3	11.8 ± 7.1
Old adult	6.6 ± 3.0	24.6 ± 12.3
Upper inner arm		
Young adult	12.2 ± 5.5	14.0 ± 6.0
Old adult	6.2 ± 3.2	24.1 ± 9.5

Note: All values are Mean ± S.D. for 12 young or 12 old subjects. Young (<30 years) and old (>65 years) groups differ from each other in both sites for both parameters ($p < .02$). Two individuals who failed to blister were assigned a value of 60 min.

allergens fell from 53% at age 20 years to 16% at age 75 years.[22] The smaller group of subjects with at least three, seven, or eleven positive tests showed parallel reductions with advancing adult age. The investigators were unable to determine the relative contributions of systemic vs. local cutaneous changes in this decline.

In another study of 740 patients reporting a prior penicillin-induced urticarial eruption, appropriate percutaneous and interdermal skin testing produced a positive wheal reaction in 69% of those under 30 years of age, but in only 39% of those older than 30 years.[66] The authors note that this discrepancy might be due to the older patients' longer average interval between their clinical reaction and testing, a second variable that statistically influenced the prevalence of positive tests, rather than a true age-related inability to respond.

F. Vitamin D Production

An endocrine function of human skin suspected to decline with age is vitamin D production. In response to UVB or solar irradiation, both the epidermis and dermis convert 7-dehydro-cholesterol to previtamin D_3, which then undergoes spontaneous conversion to vitamin D_3.[67] Because of intrinsic tissue capacity[68] and the limited penetration of the responsible wavelengths into human skin,[6] this reaction occurs principally in the epidermis. Vitamin D_3 is then bound to a specific carrier protein, transported into the circulation, and subsequently hydroxylated by both the liver and kidneys to its biological active form 1,25-$(OH)_2$-vitamin D, which acts on multiple tissues to regulate calcium metabolism.[69] With advancing age, bone mass decreases markedly, especially in postmenopausal women, predisposing to trabecular bone fractures.[70] Osteoporosis, or lack of cortical and trabecular bone, is a prominent factor, but recent studies have demonstrated that many elderly individuals also have osteomalacia, decreased mineralization of bone, classically associated with vitamin D deficiency. In the U.K., where dietary supplementation with vitamin D has been discontinued, 20 to 30% of women and up to 40% of men with femoral fractures have occult osteomalacia as determined by bone biopsy;[71-73] and in one study[74] approximately 25% of elderly American patients hospitalized with intracapsular hip fractures also had histologic evidence of osteomalacia, despite the availability of dietary supplements. Furthermore, a survey of representative elderly nursing home residents in the Boston area revealed that 25 to 30% of these asymptomatic individuals had serologic evidence of vitamin D deficiency.[98] Although avoidence of dairy products, the principal dietary source of vitamin D, and insufficient sun exposure undoubtedly contribute to vitamin D deficiency in the elderly, Holick and coworkers have recently determined that the level of epidermal 7-dehydrocholesterol per unit skin surface area decreases linearly by approximately 75% between early and late adulthood (18 to 85 years)[75] suggesting that lack of the immediate biosynthetic precursor may also limit vitamin D production. This possible age-associated functional deficiency of human skin warrants careful investigation, since bone fractures are a major cause of morbidity and mortality in the elderly.

IV. BIOCHEMICAL AND BIOPHYSICAL CHANGES

Published studies of age-associated biochemical and biophysical changes in the skin are virtually restricted to the dermis, frequently involve nonhuman tissue, and in some instances fail to control for the effects of chronic solar irradiation. In addition, the changes in collagen, elastin, and ground substances which have been described during fetal and early postnatal development are far greater than those which have been described with advancing age during adulthood. Much of the published work relies on methodology available for more than a decade and is well reviewed elsewhere.[1,2,76]

Recent work on aging in collagen confirms a slight but progressive increase in the force of contraction (isometric tension) on rat tail tendon heated above its shrinkage temperature, consistent with increasing cross-linkage of the collagen molecule.[77,78] Others have previously shown a progressive decrease in the ratio of soluble to insoluble collagen in both rat tail tendon[79] and human skin.[80-82] The predominant cross-links in skin, hydroxy-, and dihydroxylysinonorleucine, have been reported to decrease and virtually disappear with age in mature animals, however, using techniques which measure borohydride-reducible cross-links,[78] despite evidence of increasing mechanical stability. This suggests that with age collagen may form progressive cross-links which are then reduced or oxidized in vivo, and are therefore not measurable (Figure 10).

The proportion of recently synthesized human dermal collagen as determined by neutral salt extraction is small and does not vary with age in adults.[84,85] However, there is a significant decrease with age in the percent of total collagen that is released by pepsin digestion and hence incompletely cross-linked, from approximately 25% at age 30 years to approximately 10% at age 75 years, with a proportionate increase in the percent of insoluble collagen from approximately 70 to 88%.[85] The amount of ketoamine-linked glycosylation of insoluble dermal collagen also increases with age,[85] possibly related to slower collagen turnover or higher average glucose levels in the tissue. Elastin fibers in skin are less well studied, but have been reported to show progressive cross-linkage and calcification with age in adult skin.[86]

Prolyl and lysyl hydroxylase, enzymes necessary for intercellular stabilization of the collagen triple helix and for its intermolecular cross-linking, show an age-associated decline in activity in human skin,[87,88] primarily during the fetal and postnatal development period, although these enzyme activities in cultured dermal fibroblasts from donors ranging in age from a few months to 94 years do not.[89] This apparent contradiction could be explained by an age-associated decrease in either dermal fibroblast number in vivo or in fibroblast responsiveness to a serum-derived enzyme stimulating factor.[89]

There are few data concerning the possible postmaturational age-associated changes in mucopolysaccharides (glycosaminoglycans and proteoglycans) or other molecules of the ground substances in which collagen and elastic fibers are embedded. There appears to be a slight decrease with age in mucopolysaccharide content relative to dry weight or collagen content of the skin,[90-92] especially for hyaluronic acid.[92] Although mucopolysaccharides constitute only 0.1 to 0.3% of dry weight for whole skin,[93] this decrease may adversely influence skin turgor, as proteolycans "bind" a volume of water in the dermis up to 1000 times the size of the molecule itself.[94] In addition, mucopolysaccharides influence migration, growth and differentiation of connective tissue cells in at least some instances.[95]

Mechanical properties of the skin also change with age during adulthood. Uniaxial and biaxial tension tests performed on excised abdominal skin strips were reported to demonstrate progressive loss of elastic recovery, consistent with gradual destruction of the dermal elastin network, although few data were presented.[96] In the same paper, the time required for excised skin to return to its original thickness after 50% compression for 10 min was markedly prolonged in elderly vs. young adults. In the young specimens approximately 90% recovery occurred within 2 to 3 min while in the old specimens, recovery at 20 min was still below 70%.[96] Measuring changes in weight and volume after application of negative pressure to mouse tail or ear specimens, other investigators have determined that edema induced by a standardized stimulus is less in old adult than in young adult animals,[97] probably because of the age-associated decrease in vascular surface area.

Overall, a picture emerges of aging dermis as an increasingly rigid, inelastic tissue, less capable of undergoing either biochemical or mechanical modification in response to stress.

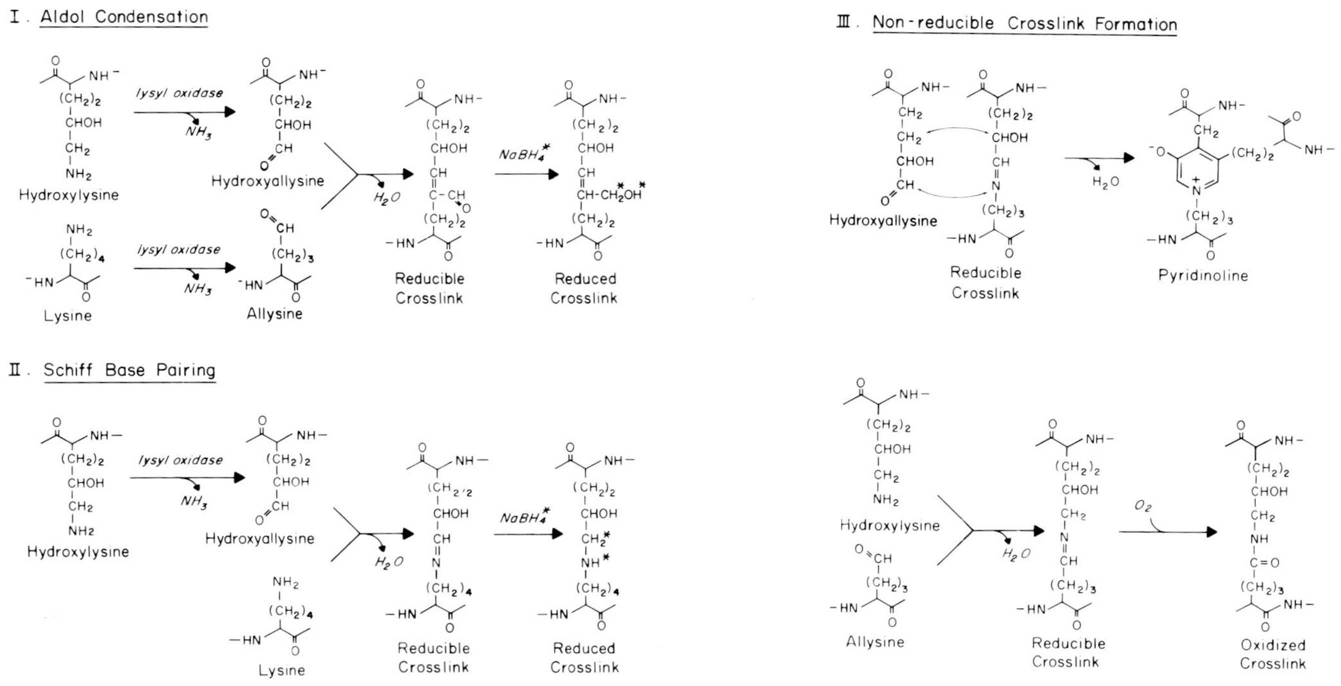

FIGURE 10. Postulated age-associated collagen cross-linkages. In the above sequence, intermolecular and intramolecular cross-links are formed between adjacent collagen chains by either aldol condensation or Schiff base pairing. Hydroxylysine and lysine may cross-link with either of their deaminated products, hydroxyallysine or allysine, a total of eight possible combinations. These cross-links are stable, but may be reduced by addition of radiolabeled sodium borohydride (NaB_4*) in order to quantify the number of cross-links by measuring the amount of tritiated reaction product. With increasing age, however, tritium incorporation into collagen following reaction with $NaBH_4*$ decreases despite biophysical evidence of increasing cross-linkage.[78] This suggests that during aging the reactive double bonds may be reduced in vivo by one or both of the mechanisms shown in the lower portion of the figure. The possible formation of pyridinoline is especially intriguing, as this compound fluoresces[83] and may therefore account for the increasing dermal fluorescence noted with age in human skin. (Schema modified from Irene Kochevar, Ph.D., oral presentation, and the indicated references.)

REFERENCES

1. **Montagna, W.,** *Advances in the Biology of Skin,* Vol. 6, Aging, Pergamon Press, Oxford, 1965, 273.
2. **Selmanowitz, V. J., Rizer, R. L., and Orentreich, N.,** Aging of the skin and its appendages, in *Handbook of the Biology of Aging,* Finch, C. E. and Hayflick, L., Eds., Van Nostrand Rheinhold Co., New York, 1977, 496.
3. **Montagna, W., Kligman, A. M., Wuepper, K. D., and Bentley, J. P.,** Special issue on aging. Proceedings of the 28th Symposium on the Biology of the Skin, *J. Invest. Dermatol.,* 73, 1, 1979.
4. **Gilchrest, B. A.,** Some gerontologic considerations in the practice of dermatology, *Arch. Dermatol.,* 115, 1343, 1979.
5. **Rowe, J. W.,** Clinical research on aging: strategies and directions, *N. Engl. J. Med.,* 297, 1332, 1977.
6. **Parrish, J. A., Anderson, R. R., Urbach, F., and Pitts, D.,** *UVA: Biological Effects of Ultraviolet Radiation with Emphasis on Human Response to Longwave Ultraviolet,* Plenum Press, New York, 1978.
7. **Hill, W. R. and Montgomery, H.,** Regional changes and changes caused by age in the normal skin, *J. Invest. Dermatol.,* 3, 321, 1940.
8. **Montagna, W. and Carlisle, K.,** Structural changes in aging human skin, *J. Invest. Dermatol.,* 73, 47, 1979.
9. **Anderson, W., Behnke, R. H., and Sato, T.,** Changes with advancing age in the cell population of human dermis, *Gerontologia,* 10, 1, 1965.
9a. **Katzberg, A. K.,** The area of the dermo-epidermal junction in human skin, *Anat. Record,* 131, 717, 1958.
10. **Montagna, W.,** Morphology of the aging skin: the cutaneous appendages, in *Advances in the Biology of the Skin,* Vol. 6, Aging, Montagna, W., Ed., Pergamon Press, Oxford, 1965, 1.
11. **Lavker, R. M.,** Structural alterations in exposed and unexposed aged skin, *J. Invest Dermatol.,* 73, 59, 1979.
12. **Lavker, R. M., Kwong, F., and Kligman, A. M.,** Changes in skin surface patterns with age, *J. Gerontol.,* 35, 348, 1980.
13. **Fitzpatrick, T. B., Szabo, G., and Mitchell, R.,** Age changes in the human melanocyte system, in *Advances in the Biology of the Skin,* Vol. 6, Aging, Montagna, W., Ed., Pergamon Press, Oxford, 1965, 35.
14. **Quevado, W. C., Jr., Szabo, G., and Vicks, J.,** Influences of age and UV on the population of dopa-positive melanocytes in human skin, *J. Invest. Dermatol.,* 52, 287, 1969.
15. **Gilchrest, B. A., Blog, F. B., and Szabo, G.,** The effect of aging and chronic ultraviolet irradiation on melanocytes in human skin, *J. Invest. Dermatol.,* 52, 141, 1979.
16. **Maize, J. C. and Foster, G.,** Age-related changes in melanocytic nevi, *Clin. Exp. Dermatol.,* 4, 49, 1979.
17. Special issue on dendritic and lymphocytic cells in the epidermis, *J. Invest. Dermatol.,* 75, 1, 1980.
18. **Gilchrest, B. A., Murphy, G., and Soter, N. A.,** Effects of chronologic aging and ultraviolet irradiation on Langerhans cells in human skin, *J. Invest. Dermatol.,* 79, 85, 1982.
19. **Black, M. M.,** A modified radiographic method for measuring skin thickness, *Br. J. Dermatol.,* 81, 661, 1969.
20. **Tan, C. Y., Statham, B., Marks, R., and Payne, P. A.,** Skin thickness measurement by pulsed ultrasound: its reproducibility, validation and variability, *Br. J. Dermatol.,* 106, 657, 1982.
21. **Gilchrest, B. A., Stoff, J. S., and Soter, N. A.,** Chronologic aging alters the response to UV-induced inflammation in human skin, *J. Invest. Dermatol.,* 79, 11, 1982.
22. **Barbee, R. A., Lebowitz, M. D., Thompson, H. C., and Burrows, B.,** Immediate skin-test reactivity in a general population sample, *Ann. Intern. Med.,* 84, 129, 1976.
23. **Azizkhan, K. G., Azizkhan, J. C., Zetter, B. R., and Folkman, J.,** Mast cell heparin stimulates migration of capillary endothelial cells in vitro, *J. Exp. Med.,* 152, 931, 1980.
24. **Kligman, A. M.,** Perspectives and problems in cutaneous gerontology, *J. Invest. Dermatol.,* 73, 39, 1979.
25. **Braverman, I. M. and Fonferko, E.,** Studies in cutaneous aging. I. The elastic fiber network, *J. Invest. Dermatol.,* 78, 434, 1982.
26. **Braverman, I. M. and Fonferko, E.,** Studies in cutaneous aging. II. The microvasculature, *J. Invest. Dermatol.,* 78, 444, 1982.
27. **Giacometti, L.,** The anatomy of the human scalp, in *Advances in the Biology of the Skin,* Vol. 6, Aging, Montagna, W., Ed., Pergamon Press, Oxford, 1965, 97.
28. **Oberste-Lehn, H.,** Effects of aging on the papillary body of the hair follicles and on the eccrine sweat glands, in *Advances in the Biology of the Skin,* Vol. 6, Aging, Montagna, W., Ed., Pergamon Press, Oxford, 1965, 17.
29. **Keogh, E. V. and Walsh, R. J.,** Rate of greying of human hair, *Nature (London),* 207, 877, 1965.
30. **Burch, P. R. J., Murray, J. J., and Jackson, D.,** The age-prevalence of arcus senilis, greying of hair, and baldness. Etiological considerations, *J. Gerontol.,* 26, 364, 1971.

31. **Barman, J. M., Percoraro, V., and Astore, I.,** Biological bases of the inception and evolution of baldness, *J. Gerontol.,* 24, 163, 1969.

32. **Hanna, M. and MacMillan, A. L.,** The skin, in *Aging and the Skin,* Brocklehurst, J. C., Ed., Churchill Livingstone, Edinburgh and London, 1973, 593.

33. **Cawley, E. P., Hsu, Y. T., Sturgill, B. C., and Harman, L. E.,** Lipofuscin ("wear and tear" pigment) in human sweat glands, *J. Invest. Dermatol.,* 61, 105, 1973.

34. **Winkelmann, R. K.,** Nerve changes in aging skin, in *Advances in the Biology of the Skin,* Vol. 6, Aging, Montagna, W., Ed., Pergamon Press, Oxford, 1965, 51.

35. **Meissner, G.** *Beitraege zur Anatomie und Physiologie der Haut,* Leopold Voss, Leipzig, 1853, 22.

36. **Rongue, H.,** Altersveranderungen der meissnerschen korperchen in der fingerhaut, A mikr-anat, *Forsch,*54, 167, 1943.

37. **Cauna, N.,** The effects of aging on the receptor organs of the human dermis, in *Advances in the Biology of the Skin,* Vol. 6, Aging, Montagna, W., Ed., Pergamon Press, Oxford, 1965, 63.

38. **Leyden, J. J., McGinley, K. J., and Grove, G. L.,** Age-related differences in the rate of desquamation of skin surface cells, in *Pharmacological Intervention in the Aging Process,* Adelman, R. D., Roberts, J., and Cristofalo, V. J., Eds., Plenum Press, New York, 1978, 297.

39. **Grove, G. L. and Kligman, A. M.,** Age-associated changes in human epidermal cell renewal, *J. Gerontol.,* 38, 137, 1983.

40. **Baker, H. and Blair, C. P.,** Cell replacement in the human stratum corneum in old age, *Br. J. Dermatol.,* 80, 367, 1967.

41. **Orentreich, N., Markofsky, J., and Vogelman, J. H.,** The effect of aging on the rate of linear nail growth, *J. Invest. Dermatol.,* 73, 126, 1979.

42. **Sandblom, P. H., Petersen, P., and Muren, A.,** Determination of the tensile strength of healing wounds as a clinical test, *Acta Cher. Scand.,* 105, 252, 1953.

43. **Viljanto, J. A.,** A sponge implant method for testing connective tissue regeneration in surgical patients, *Acta Cher. Scand.,* 135, 297, 1969.

44. **Grove, G. L.,** Age-related differences in healing of superficial skin wounds in humans, *Arch. Dermatol. Res.,* 272, 381, 1982.

45. **Sbano, E., Andereassi, L., Fimiani, M., et al.,** DNA-repair after UV-irradiation in skin fibroblasts from patients with actinic keratosis, *Arch. Dermatol. Res.,* 262, 55, 1978.

46. **Tindall, J. P. and Smith, J. G.,** Skin lesions of the aged, *JAMA,* 186, 1039, 1963.

47. **Scotto, J., Kopf, A. W., and Urbach, F.,** Non-melanoma skin cancer among Caucasians in four areas of the United States, *Cancer,* 34, 1333, 1974.

48. **Martin, G. M.,** Proliferative hemeotasis and its age-related aberrations, *Mech. Aging Dev.,* 9, 385, 1979.

49. **Cristophers, E. and Kligman, A. M.,** Percutaneous absorption in aged skin, in *Advances in the Biology of the Skin,* Vol. 6, Aging, Montagna, W., Ed., Pergamon Press, Oxford, 1965, 163.

50. **Grove, G. L., Lavker, R. M., Hoelzle, E., and Kligman, A. M.,** Use of nonintrusive tests to monitor age-associated changes in human skin, *J. Soc. Cosmet. Chem.,* 32, 15, 1981.

50a. **Grove, G. L., Duncan, S., and Kligman, A. M.,** Effect of aging on the blistering of human skin with ammonium hydroxide, *Br. J. Dermatol.,* 107, 393, 1982.

51. **Schluderman, E. and Zubeck, J. P.,** Effect of age on pain sensitivity, *Percept. Mot. Skills,* 14, 295, 1952.

52. **Sherman, E. D. and Robillard, E.,** Sensitivity to pain in relationship to age, *J. Am. Geriatr. Soc.,* 12, 1037, 1964.

53. **Procacci, P., Bozza, G., Buzzelli, G., and Della Corte, M.,** The cutaneous pricking pain threshold in old age, *Gerontol. Clin.,* 12, 213, 1970.

54. **Procacci, P., Della Corte, M., Zoppi, M., Romano, S., Maresca, M., and Voegelin, M.,** Pain threshold measurement in man, in *Recent Advances on Pain: Pathophysiology and Clinical Aspects,* Bonica, J. J., Procacci, P., and Pagoni, C., Eds., Charles C Thomas, Springfield, Ill., 1974, 105.

55. **Kenshalo, D. R.,** Age changes in touch, vibration, temperature, kinesthesis, and pain sensitivity, in *Handbook of the Psychology of Aging,* Birren, J. E. and Schaie, K. W., Eds., Van Nostrand Reinhold, New York, 1977, 562.

56. **Melzack, R. and Casey, K. L.,** Sensory, motivational, and central control of determinants of pain, in *The Skin Senses,* Kenshalo, D. R., Ed., Charles C Thomas, Springfield, Ill., 1968, 423.

57. **Silver, A. F., Montagna, W., and Karacan, I.,** The effect of age on human eccrine sweating, in *Advances in the Biology of the Skin,* Vol. 6, Aging, Montagna, W., Ed., Pergamon Press, Oxford, 1965, 129.

58. **MacKinnon, P. C. B.,** Variations with age in the number of active palmar digital sweat glands, *J. Neurol. Neurosurg. Psych.,* 17, 124, 1954.

59. **Pochi, P. E., Strauss, J. S., and Downing, D. T.,** Age-related changes in sebaceous gland activity, *J. Invest. Dermatol.,* 73, 108, 1979.

60. **Besdine, R. W.,** Geriatric medicine: an overview, in *Annual Review of Geronotology and Geriatrics,* Eisdorfer, C., Ed., Springer Publishing Co., New York, 1979, 135.

61. **Kiistala, U.,** Dermal-epidermal separation. I. The influence of age, sex, and body region on suction blister formation in human skin, *Ann. Clin. Res.,* 4, 10, 1972.

62. **Jordon, R. E.,** Bullous pemphigoid, cicatricial pemphigoid, and chronic bullous dermatosis in childhood, in *Dermatology in General Medicine,* Fitzpatrick, T. B., Eisen, A. Z., Wolff, K., Freedberg, I. M., and Austen, K. F., Eds., McGraw-Hill, New York, 1979, 318.

63. **Walford, D. S., Willkens, R. F., and Decker, J. L.,** Impaired delayed hypersensitivity in an aging population: association with antinuclear reactivity and rheumatoid factor, *JAMA,* 203, 831, 1968.

64. **Roberts-Thomson, I. C., Whittingham, S., Youngchaiyud, U., et al.,** Aging, immune response, and mortality, *Lancet,* 2, 368, 1974.

65. **Mackay, I. R.,** Changes in human lymphocyte activity with age, *Interdiscipl. Topics Gerontol.,* 11, 75, 1977.

66. **Sullivan, T. J., Wedner, H. J., Shatz, G. S., Yecies, L. D., and Parker, C. W.,** Skin testing to detect penicillin allergy, *J. Allergy Clin. Immunol.,* 68, 171, 1981.

67. **Holick, M. F.,** The cutaneous photosynthesis of previtamin D_3: a unique photoendocrine system, *J. Invest. Dermatol.,* 76, 51, 1981.

68. **Holick, M. F., MacLaughlin, J. A., Clark, M. B., Holick, S. A., Potts, J. T., Jr., Anderson, R. R., Blank, I. H., and Parrish, J. A.,** Photosynthesis of previtamin D_3 in human skin and the physiologic consequences, *Science,* 210, 203, 1980.

69. **Holick, M. F. and Potts, J. T., Jr.,** Vitamin D, in *Harrison's Principles of Internal Medicine,* 9th ed., Isselbacher, K. J., Adams, R. D., Braunwald, E., Petersdorf, R. G., and Wilson, J. D., Eds., McGraw-Hill, New York, 1980, 1843.

70. **Nordin, B. E. C., Peacock, M., Aaron, J., Crilly, R. G., Heyburn, P. J., Horsman, A., and Marshall, D.,** Osteoporosis and osteomalacia, *Clin. Endocrinol. Metab.,* 9, 177, 1980.

71. **Exton-Smith, A. N., Hodkinson, N. M., and Stanton, E. R.,** Nutrition and metabolic bone disease in old age, *Lancet,* 2, 999, 1966.

72. **Jenkins, D. H. R., Webster, R. D., and Williams, E. O.,** Osteomalacia in elderly patients with fracture of the femoral neck, *J. Bone Jt. Surg.,* 55, 575, 1973.

73. **Anderson, T., Campbell, A. E., Dunn, A., and Runciman, J. B. M.,** Osteomalacia in elderly women, *Scot. Med. J.,* 11, 429, 1966.

74. **Sokoloff, L.,** Occult osteomalacia in American (USA) patients with fracture of the hip, *Am. J. Surg. Pathol.,* 2, 21, 1978.

75. **Holick, M. F. and MacGlaughlin, J. A.,** Aging significantly decreases the capacity of human epidermis to produce vitamin D_3, *Clin. Res.,* 408A, 1981.

76. **Kivirikko, K. I. and Pisteli, L.,** Biosynthesis of collagen and its alteration in pathological states, *Med. Biol.,* 54, 159, 1976.

77. **Bentley, J. P.,** Aging of collagen, *J. Invest. Dermatol.,* 73, 80, 1979.

78. **Allain, J. C., LeLous, N., Bazin, S., Bailey, A. J., and Delaunay, A.,** Isometric tension developed during heating of collagenous tissue-relationship with collagen cross linking, *Biochem. Biophys. Acta,* 533, 147, 1978.

79. **Cannon, D. J. and Davidson, P. F.,** Cross-linking and aging in rat tendon collagen, *Exp. Gerontol.,* 8, 51, 1973.

80. **Sams, W. M. and Smith, J. G., Jr.,** Alterations in human dermal fibrous connective tissue with age and chronic sun damage, in *Advances in the Biology of Skin,* Vol. 6, Aging, Montagna, W., Ed., Pergamon Press, Oxford, 1965, 199.

81. **Bakerman, S.,** Quantitative extraction of acid-soluble human skin collagen with age, *Nature (London),* 196, 375, 1962.

82. **Miyahara, T., Murai, A., Tanaka, T., Shiozawa, S., and Kameyama, M.,** Age-related differences in human skin collagen: solubility in solvent, susceptibility to pepsin digestion, and the spectrum of the solubilized polymeric collagen molecules, *J. Gerontol.,* 37, 651, 1982.

83. **Sakura, S., Fujimot, D., Sakamoto, K., Mizuno, A. and Motegi, K.,** Photolysis of pyridinoline, a cross-linking amino acid of collagen, by ultraviolet light, *Can. J. Biochem.,* 60, 525, 1982.

84. **Uitto, J., Øhlenschlager, K., and Lorengen, I.,** Solubility of skin collagen in normal human subjects and in patients with generalized scleroderm, *Clin. Chim. Acta,* 31, 13, 1971.

85. **Schnider, S. L. and Kohn, R. R.,** Effects of age and diabetes mellitus on the solubility and nonenzymatic glycosylation of human skin collagen, *J. Clin. Invest.,* 67, 1630, 1981.

86. **Patridge, S. M.,** Biological role of cutaneous elastin, in *Advances in the Biology of Skin,* Vol. 10, Montagna, W., Bentley, J. P., and Dobson, R. L., Eds., Meredith Corp., New York, 1970, 69.

87. **Anttinen, H., Orva, S., Ryhanen, L., and Kivirikko, K. I.,** Assay of protocollagen lysyl hydroxylase activity in the skin of human subjects and changes in the activity with age, *Clin. Chem. Acta,* 47, 289, 1973.

88. **Tuderman, L. and Kivirikko, K. I.,** Immuno-reactive prolyl hydroxylase in human skin, serum, and synovial fluid: changes in the content and components with age, *Eur. J. Clin. Invest.,* 7, 295, 1977.

89. **Musad, S., Sivarajah, A., and Pinnell, S. R.,** Prolyl and lysyl hydroxylase activities of human skin fibroblasts: effect of donor age and ascorbate, *J. Invest. Dermatol.,* 75, 404, 1980.

90. **Clausen, B.,** Influence of age on chondroitin sulfates and collagen of human aorta, myocardium, and skin, *Lab Invest.,* 12, 538, 1963.

91. **Breen, M., et al.,** Acidic lycosaminoglycans in human skin during fetal development and adult life, *Biochim. Biophys. Acta,* 201, 54, 1970.

92. **Fleischmajer, R., et al.,** Human dermal glycosaminoglycans and aging, *Biochim. Biophys. Acta,* 279, 265, 1972.

93. **Pearce, R. H.,** Glycosaminoglycans and glycoproteins in skin, in *The Amino Sugars,* Balazs, E.A. and Jeanloz, R. W., Eds., Academic Press, New York, 1965, 149.

94. **Silbert, J. E.,** Mucopolysaccharides of ground substances, in *Dermatology in General Medicine,* Fitzpatrick, T. B., Eisen, A. Z., Wolff, K., Freedberg, I. M., and Austen, K. F., Eds., McGraw-Hill, New York, 1979, 189.

95. **Toole, B. P.,** Morphogenetic role of glycosaminoglycans (acid mucopolysaccharides) in brain and other tissue, in *Neural Recognition,* Barondes, S., Ed., Plenum Press, New York, 1976, 275.

96. **Daly, C. H. and Odland, G. F.,** Age-related changes in the mechanical properties of human skin, *J. Invest. Dermatol.,* 73, 84, 1979.

97. **Rosenthal, S. M. and LaJohn, L. A.,** Effect of age on transvascular fluid movement, *Am. J. Physiol.,* 228, 134, 1975.

98. **Holick, M. F.,** personal communication.

Chapter 4

PATHOLOGIC PROCESSES IN THE SKIN ASSOCIATED WITH AGING

I. INTRODUCTION

No skin disease occurs exclusively in the elderly, but some disorders do occur more commonly in this age group. Moreover, the same conditions may evolve differently in older patients and treatment regimens derived from experience with young adults may require modification to ensure optimal efficacy and safety.

Although some age-specific incidence and prevalence figures are available, there are very few data concerning age-associated qualitative changes in the presentation and response to therapy for these skin diseases. This chapter briefly reviews several dermatologic disorders relevant to the elderly and attempts to emphasize those diagnostic and therapeutic issues that may be influenced by patient age.

II. DECUBITUS ULCERS

The decubitus ulcer or pressure sore is one of the most difficult management problems encountered in geriatric patients and is common among those confined to bed or wheelchair. The lesion is better classified as a systemic rather than cutaneous disorder, as major illness involving at least one and usually several organ systems is invariably present. Indeed, decubitus ulcers are a major problem in clinical medicine precisely because the predisposing factors are of paramount importance and rarely correctable.

The ulcers occur over bony prominences: statistically 65% in the pelvic area and 30% on the lower extremities.[1] Prolonged direct pressure, in excess of the 32 mmHg average capillary perfusion pressure in the skin, produces tissue anoxia with necrosis of epidermis and superficial dermis. Since pressure up to 70 mmHg may be generated at the sacrum and 45 mmHg at the heels when the body is supine, it is not surprising that decubitus ulcers may arise after as little as an hour of total immobility. Additional contributing factors in the elderly often include: (1) folding of loose lax skin with compromised blood flow in larger dermal vessels as well as increased compression of superficial capillaries, (2) reduced subcutaneous fat which results in greater local pressure on the skin over bony prominence such as the ischial tuberosities and sacrum, and (3) reduction in baseline cutaneous blood flow by congestive heart failure, atherosclerosis, loss of intravascular volume, or other disorders common in advanced age.

Local factors leading to the development of decubitus ulcers have been explored further in an important recent study,[2] the first to actually obtain pressure readings in frail elderly as well as healthy young adults. Fourteen hospitalized geriatric patients without decubitus ulcers were compared to nine young control subjects. External pressure, shear, and blood flow in the ischial area were measured with subjects sitting in a specially equipped wheelchair. The external pressure necessary for complete blood flow cessation exceeded 120 mmHg in all the young subjects, but ranged from less than 20 mmHg in two elderly subjects to 150 mmHg in one, with a much reduced average value for the elderly group. Older patients also manifested much greater variation in pressure over the sitting surface. This implies that an older individual experiences foci of greater pressure when seated or lying on a firm surface than does a younger individual of the same size and weight, possibly due to loss of skin "tone," that property of the dermis responsible for conducting forces away from local maxima in young adult skin. Shear forces generated largely by folding and lateral displacement of lax skin, were three times greater in the elderly than in the young. Not surprisingly, at any given external presure, the elderly were far more likely to experience vascular occlusion. The investigators also observed that tipping the chair seat back greatly reduced pressure and shear over the ischial tuberosities in the elderly subjects, but did not alter the pressure in the young; pressure over the sacrum was not measured during the procedure.

Once a decubitus ulcer forms, healing may be retarded by general inanition, by incontinence with secondary chemical irritation and bacterial contamination of the ulcer base, or by inadequate vascular supply of the involved area. These same factors are responsible for the inexorable progression of many decubitus ulcers into the underlying fat, muscle, and ultimately bone.

Prevention, although difficult in high risk patients, is much easier than cure. All effective measures redistribute pressure from bony prominences. The simplest is frequent turning of the bedridden patient, at least every 2 hr. Air-space or fluid-filled mattresses tend to equalize pressure over the entire area of contact and are thus a major improvement over conventional mattresses. Strategically placed pillows are theoretically helpful, but in practice rarely remain in place for long periods. Undoubtedly the best of the currently available support surfaces is the ripple mattress, a series of contiguous, 12-cm diameter horizontally aligned inflatable tubes. A machine pump repeatedly inflates and deflates the tubes every 5 to 10 min in an alternating pattern, so that the patient is supported first by the even-numbered tubes, then by the odd-numbered tubes, and no area is continuously weight bearing for more than the 5 to 10-min pump cycle time.

Once a decubitus ulcer is present, in addition to the above measures it is necessary to maintain the ulcer base in as optimal condition for healing as possible. Surgical debridement of necrotic tissue may be necessary initially. If an eschar is present, it should be removed in order to permit reepithelialization. Healing is always slowed by heavy colonization of the ulcer with bacteria, the species depending on body site, patient continence, and recent antibiotic administration. Frequent changes of wet-to-dry saline dressings, at least four times daily, provide gentle debridement and substantially reduce bacterial counts. Routine use of systemic antibiotics is ill-advised, since tissue levels are often subtherapeutic in the ulcer bed when sufficient elsewhere to dangerously alter bowel and skin flora. Topical antibiotics also penetrate granulation tissue poorly, may have a direct adverse effect on wound healing, and occasionally induce marked allergic sensitization with its attendant discomfort and risk of cross-reaction to subsequently administered systemic drugs. Antibiotic usage may be justified for 2 to 3 days preceding definitive surgical treatment of a decubitus ulcer, however, as the probability of a successful closure falls from greater than 90% to less than 20% when bacterial counts exceed 10^5/g of tissue. The choice of antibiotics should ideally be based on a recent culture of granulation tissue excised from the ulcer crater. Acetic acid 0.25 to 1.0% solution applied as a wet-to-dry dressing is especially helpful for pseudomonas organisms; other agents are usually best given by the intramuscular or intravenous route.

Mixtures of trypsin, streptokinase, vitamin E, dextran polymers, estrogens, and androgens are among the other agents intended to speed healing of decubitus ulcers, but the experience with them is almost entirely anecdotal and uncontrolled.

Maintaining a positive nitrogen balance with a normal serum protein level is undeniably beneficial, and may require supplementary feedings via naso-gastric tube or intravenous hyperalimentation line. Deficiencies of ascorbic acid and zinc, both implicated in wound healing, should be corrected if present.

Finally, surgical closure of decubitus ulcers is often preferable to the extremely slow process of natural healing. Primary closure, grafting, or rotation of a skin flap are excellent procedures in appropriate patients.

III. XEROSIS

Xerosis, the term used to describe the "dry" or rough quality of skin that is almost universal among the elderly, is a misnomer. The condition may be generalized, but is especially prominent on the lower legs and is exacerbated by low humidity environments classically found in overheated rooms during cold weather.

Xerosis probably reflects minor abnormalities in the epidermal maturation process that in turn result in an irregular surface for the stratum corneum; to date it has not been investigated experimentally. The initial assumption that the disorder resulted from a lack of water in the skin has been disproven by several investigators.[3,4] Water content of abdominal skin has been reported to increase slightly, although not statistically, from a mean value of 58% in the fourth decade to 63% in the ninth decade; while the rate of diffusional water loss across the stratum corneum in vivo appears constant with age.[3] The occasional classification of xerosis as a disorder of sebaceous (oil) glands[5] is similarly without experimental basis. Furthermore, "dry skin" in the elderly is probably quite different from "dry skin" in children and young adults, a disorder akin to mild eczematous dermatitis and often responsive to topical steroid therapy.

Whatever its etiology, xerotic skin in the elderly is often pruritic and may show evidence of inflammation, probably due to defects in the stratum corneum with secondary entry of irritating substances into the dermis. the resulting condition, called erythema craquele or winter eczema, responds promptly to topical cortiocosteroid ointment and/or emollients, although these preparations do not correct the xerosis itself (Plate 1).*

"Dry skin" is best treated prophylactically by avoidance of sun-exposure and other cumulative injuries ultimately reflected in abnormal epidermal maturation. Once xerosis is present, frequent regular use of a topical emollient makes the skin more attractive and more comfortable and prevents the complications discussed above.

The mechanism of action of emollients is so poorly understood by most physicians and virtually all patients and so misrepresented by current advertisements that some discussion is warranted. Figure 1 schematically represents normal, "dry," and treated "dry" skin. In normal skin, there is an orderly progression of keratinocytes from the viable epidermis to the overlying stratum corneum (SC). The morphologic transition occurs abruptly, immediately above the granular layer, although the process of terminal differentiation is gradual. The keratinocytes or corneocytes in the SC are flattened discs composed of keratin proteins, enclosed by permeable cross-linked protein envelopes. The water content is quite low, dropping abruptly from approximately 70% in the viable granular layer, in equilibrium with the rest of the internal milieu, to near zero at the skin surface. The number of cell layers in the SC is similar to that in epidermis, approximately 7 to 5 in most sites under normal conditions, and the corneocytes are arranged in an orderly fashion parallel to the skin surface. The result is skin which looks and feels smooth. In "dry skin" the situation differs in that the corneocyte arrangement is less orderly, with many cells disposed at an angle to the surface; the water content of the viable epidermis and the water gradient within the SC are normal. The rather rigid disc-like corneocytes projecting from the skin surface refract incident light unevenly, causing a scaly or dull appearance, and feel rough to touch. Immersing the skin in water rapidly hydrates the SC and causes individual corneocytes to swell. Corneocyte edges are thus rounded, and the skin surface is smoother. However, in a low humidity environment the SC quickly loses this water by evaporation, restoring the original morphology. Repeated cycles of hydration and dehydration further disrupt the cutaneous barrier and induce "chapping." Water loss from the SC can be slowed markedly by application of a greasy (hydrophobic) substance to the surface. This is the function of an emollient. From

* Plate 1 appears after page 100.

A   B   C   D

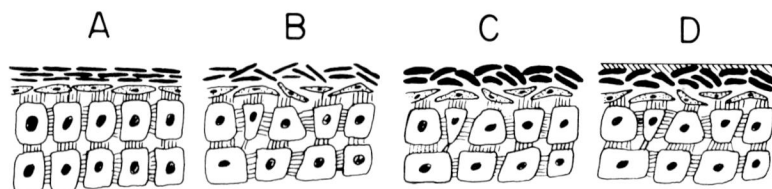

FIGURE 1.   Schematic representation of normal, ''dry'', and treated ''dry'' skin. (A) Normal skin. Note disc-like corneocytes in parallel array at the skin surface above the granular and Malpighian layers. (B) ''Dry'' skin. Corneocytes are irregularly aligned, with many cells projecting above the skin surface, reflecting disturbed maturation below. (C) ''Dry'' skin after immersion in water. Corneocytes are swollen, lacking sharp projections. There is virtually no change in the viable epidermis. (D) ''Dry'' skin after immersion in water and topical application of an emollient. A hydrophobic film overlies the swollen corneocytes, slowing water loss and further smoothing the surface.

Table 1
PRURITIC DERMATOSES THAT MAY
PRESENT AS GENERALIZED PRURITUS

Scabies	Miliaria
Atopic dermatitis (eczema)	Contact dermatitis
Dermatitis herpetiformis	Urticaria (hives)
Fiberglass dermatitis	Pediculosis
Bullous pemphigoid	

the above considerations, it is clear that emollients are most effective when applied to already moistened skin, e.g., immediately after the bath or shower. Emollients applied to nonhydrated skin act by trapping within the SC the water constantly entering it from below. However, transepidermal water loss is a slow process, and emollients have frequently worn off the skin surface before hydration is complete. ''Heavy,'' frankly greasy, emollients have the additional property of perceptibly coating the skin, producing a smooth surface film, and are usually better barriers against evaporation than are more cosmetically elegant preparations. Finally, it should be noted that emollients applied to the skin immediately after bathing retain water more effectively than gels or oils added directly to the bath water; and that such additives may coat the bathtub as well as the skin, producing a dangerously slippery and difficult-to-clean surface.

IV. PRURITUS

Elderly persons often experience localized or generalized pruritus. For some, it is a minor annoyance; for others the pruritus leads to extensive slow-healing excoriations or loss of sleep with associated irritability and impaired mental function.

Many patients presenting to the physician because of pruritus in fact have an eruption that is responsible for the symptoms, although its other manifestations may be so subtle that the patient or even the physician does not notice the rash.[6-8] Table 1 lists dermatoses that may be inconspicuous but severely pruritic. Because cutaneous inflammatory responses may be muted in the elderly,[9] a careful history and physical examination are necessary before excluding these primary disorders of the skin. Proper identification of a causative dermatoses not only leads to effective treatment in most patients,[10] but also avoids the hematologic, radiographic, and other laboratory procedures that constitute the work-up for unexplained generalized pruritus.

Table 2 lists the systemic disorders associated with generalized pruritus. Among all patients

Table 2
SYSTEMIC DISORDERS SOMETIMES ASSOCIATED WITH PRURITUS IN THE ELDERLY

Renal	Chronic renal failure
Hepatic	Extrahepatic biliary obstruction
	Hepatitis
	Drug ingestion
Hematopoietic	Polycythemia vera
	Hodgkin's disease
	Other lymphomas & leukemias
	Multiple myeloma
	Iron deficiency anemia
Endocrine	Hyperthyroidism
	Diabetes mellitus
Miscellaneous	Visceral malignancies
	Opiate ingestion
	Drug ingestion
	Psychosis

Modified and reproduced with permission from Gilchrest, B. A., *Arch. Int. Med.*, 142, 101, 1982, copyright 1982, American Medical Association.

seeking medical attention for pruritus, the prevalence of underlying systemic disease has been reported as 10 to 50%,[7,11] the percentage depending on patient selection, diagnostic evaluation, and period of follow-up.

Numerically, perhaps the most important known cause of persistent generalized pruritus is chronic renal failure. Since the inception of maintenance hemodialysis in the 1960s, survival of uremic patients has greatly increased and, with it, the prevalence of pruritus in this population. The minimum degree of renal failure necessary to cause pruritus is unknown, however, complicating interpretation of pruritus in the elderly patient with mild to moderate renal insufficiency. From a practical viewpoint, it is probably unwise to attribute pruritus to otherwise asymptomatic renal failure, or equivalently, to renal insufficiency not requiring specific therapy for any metabolic imbalance.

Pruritus is probably the most distressing and consistent symptom of chronic cholestasis, which underlies all the hepatic disorders listed in the table. Overall, pruritus occurs in approximately 20 to 25% of jaundiced patients,[12] but it is rare in those lacking cholestasis. Of special relevance to the elderly, extrahepatic biliary obstruction is often associated with pruritus. For example, in one series of 38 patients with carcinoma of the ampulla of Vater, 19 initially were seen with pruritus.[13] Drugs that can cause pruritus by inducing cholestasis include phenothiazines, tolbutamide, erythromycin estrolate, anabolic hormones, estrogens, and progestins.[14]

Approximately 30 to 50% of patients with polycythemia vera experience pruritus[15,16] classically exacerbated by hot baths, and up to 30% of patients with Hodgkin's disease also are affected.[17,18] In one recent report describing 99 patients with Hodgkin's disease, all who experienced severe pruritus did less well than stage-matched nonpruritic patients.[19] A similarly adverse effect of pruritus on disease outcome has been suggested for patients with mycosis fungoides,[20] a T-cell lymphoma primarily manifested in the skin. The incidence and significance of pruritus in other lymphomas and leukemia are unknown, but the occasional association cannot be disputed.[17] Generalized pruritus has been reported as an initial symptom in two patients with multiple myeloma and in one with Walderstrom's macroglobulinemia,[21] as well as in several with benign gammopathies.[21,22] Iron deficiency anemia has been reported as the cause of generalized pruritus in more than 50 patients by four different groups of investigators,[23,24] although this phenomenon is apparently rare.

Generalized pruritus is said to occur in 4 to 11% of patients with thyrotoxicosis, especially Graves' disease, and is probably more common in patients with long-standing untreated disease.[25] Long-standing unrecognized and hence untreated thyrotoxicosis may occur in the elderly because of the atypical presentation in this age group,[26] although the incidence of pruritus in this group is not commented upon in the literature. The pruritus occasionally associated with hypothyroidism seems to be associated with the accompanying xerosis rather than the endocrine disorder itself.

Diabetes mellitus is a frequently quoted but poorly documented cause of generalized pruritus; the least anecdotal data derive from a survey of 500 patients in 1927, in which approximately 3% reported generalized pruritus at some time after diagnosis of their diabetes.[27] There are no recent publications on the subject. In contrast, pruritus vulvae and pruritus ani secondary to Candida albicans infection are indisputably common among diabetics.[28]

Generalized pruritus may occur rarely in association with adenocarcinoma and squamous cell carcinoma of many viscera.[7,29] Opiate ingestion can provoke generalized pruritus through a central mechanism[30] or by degranulation of mast cells peripherally.[31] Other drugs may rarely cause pruritus without a rash as a manifestation of allergic sensitization.[6,7]

Psychotic persons occasionally suffer from severe generalized pruritus for which no cause is apparent; many of these patients have delusions of parasitosis.[32]

Finally, many elderly persons, up to 30% in one English survey,[33] experience generalized pruritus for which there is no apparent explanation, and one must either accept a higher incidence of idiopathic pruritus with advancing age or infer the existence of an entity "senile pruritus," the result perhaps of age-associated degenerative changes in peripheral nerve endings.

The pathophysiology of pruritus associated with these systemic diseases is incompletely understood.[34] Optimal therapy for generalized pruritus is that for the underlying disease, whenever possible. Unfortunately, the responsible disorder is either uncorrectable, or, indeed, undetectable.

In two instances, specific and often effective therapies are available for pruritic patients. Subtotal parathyroidectomy,[35,36] intravenous lidocaine,[37] UV-B irradiation,[38,39] oral cholestyramine resin,[40] and oral charcoal[41] have all benefited a majority of reported cases of uremic pruritus. Oral cholestyramine resin[42-44] and plasma perfusion using charcoal-coated beads[45] have lessened pruritus in patients with hepatobiliary disease.

For those patients whose pruritus is not amenable to the previously mentioned measures, nonspecific therapies must be employed. Often it is worthwhile to prescribe an emollient even in the absence of clinical xerosis, as minimal or intermittent dryness, present in virtually all elderly individuals, may notably exacerbate pruritus of another cause. Topical application of menthol, 0.25 to 0.5%, or the anesthetic phenol, 0.5 to 1.0%, in an appropriate vehicle also may provide considerable temporary relief; other topical anesthetics can be used only at the risk of allergic sensitization.[46] Oral antihistamines are widely prescribed for pruritus of all causes, although their efficacy is slight in most instances,[46] even when combinations of H_1 and H_2 blockers are used.[47] Antihistamines may have the additional problems in the elderly of paradoxical restlessness or significantly impaired psychomotor function.[48]

Treatment of pruritus is often unsatisfactory, especially in those patients without associated systemic disease. More effective approaches to this common and distressing symptom await a better understanding of its pathogenesis.

V. HERPES ZOSTER

Herpes zoster or "shingles" is a familiar vesicular dermatomal eruption due to reactivation of a latent varicella virus in the dorsal sensory ganglia of a partially immune host. More than two-thirds of cases occur in patients older than 50 years[49-53] with age-adjusted annual incidence rate per 1000 population less than 1 at age 0 to 10 years, approximately 2.5 at age 20 to 50 years, and more than 10 at age 80 years.[50] It has been estimated that by age 85, an individual has a 50% risk of having had at least one attack of herpes zoster and a 10% risk of having had two attacks.[50] Immunosuppressed patients, many of whom are elderly, have an annual incidence 20 to 100 times that of the general population and often have much more severe disease.[54-57]

Herpes zoster usually begins with dysesthesia or paresthesia of the involved dermatome. These symptoms persist for days to rarely longer than a week before the appearance of vesicles and may mimic angina, spinal cord compression, renal or biliary colic, muscle sprains, or many other disorders. Constitutional symptoms are rare in adults.[51] A few cases of pre-herpetic neuralgia, diagnosed by a rise in viral antibody titers, have resolved without the development of a cutaneous eruption.[58-60]

The rash of herpes zoster is virtually pathognomonic. Clusters of vesicles sometimes superimposed on an erythematous plaque, erupt in a dermatomonal distribution (Plate 2).* Lesions do not cross the midline, and the eruption is unilateral in at least 98% of patients, although occasional individual "disseminated" vesicles occur in up to one-third. The diagnosis of herpes virus infection may be confirmed by Tzanck stain of material scraped from the base of an intact vesicle.[61] The initially clear vesicles may become pustular or, especially in the elderly, hemorrhagic within a few days. New lesions continue to appear for several days, often progressing distally along the dermatome. Dissemination, if it is to occur, usually does so during this period. Pain and hyperesthesia are frequently prominent during the first days of the eruption although their severity is unrelated to either the risk or severity of postherpetic neuralgia in individual patients. Vesicles usually begin to crust in the second week and resolve within 4 weeks in most patients.[49] The eruption tends to persist longer and to be more severe in the elderly.[3,10] Vesicle fluid is contagious, but the attack rate (cases of varicella) in susceptible household contacts is much less than for chicken pox (primarily varicella infection).[50,62]

A. Complications of Herpes Zoster

The course of herpes zoster infection in young and old adults differ primarily in the incidence and severity of postherpetic neuralgia. This problem occurs in approximately 10% of cases overall, but is uncommon in patients less than 40 years old.[51] In one survey of 916 patients, more than half of those above 60 years old experienced pain lasting at least 1 year.[52] The increase in severity and duration of postherpetic neuralgia with age is even more marked than the increase in incidence. Persistent pain is especially common in these patients with trigeminal involvement,[52] 10 to 15% of reported cases,[49] or immunosuppression.[49]

Persistent hyperpigmentation or true scarring of involved skin are less important complications of herpes zoster that are also more common in the elderly.

Fortunately, patients with herpes zoster appear not to be at increased risk for the subsequent development of malignancy.[63]

B. Treatment for Herpes Zoster

During the acute phase of the infection, some patients require narcotic analgesics for

---

* Plate 2 appears after page 100.

adequate relief of pain. These agents should be prescribed cautiously in the elderly to avoid over-medication and adverse systemic effects (see ''Drug Reactions'' in this chapter).

Early skin lesions are best treated with local compresses of Burow's solution (1:20 in cool water) or other hypertonic soaks for 10 min 3 or 4 times daily, followed by gentle washing with Hibiclens or other antibacterial soap, to hasten drying and prevent bacterial superinfection. Topical antibiotic ointment may be applied twice daily to already crusted lesions.

Several forms of treatment have been proposed for the devastating problem of postherpetic neuralgia. The longest-standing and most readily available is systemically administered corticosteroids, first proposed more than 3 decades ago,[64] and since documented to be effective in two controlled trials.[65,66] In the more recent study,[66] 40 otherwise healthy patients at least 50 years old with early severe herpes zoster were randomly allocated to two groups of similar composition and average age (66.4 years and 68.5 years) for treatment with either prednisolone or carbmazepine (as a placebo). The eruption had been present an average of approximately 5 days in both groups before beginning therapy. Skin lesions healed significantly faster in the prednisolone group (3.65 vs. 5.25 weeks), and the incidence of postherpetic neuralgia was 15% (3 of 20) vs. 65% (13 of 20) in the control group. Pain in the three prednisolone-treated patients lasted 4 to 6 months, while in 4 of the 13 control patients pain persisted for at least 1 year. No patient in either group had viral dissemination or other major complications of therapy. The prednisolone was administered orally, 40 mg/day (equivalent to prednisone 40 mg/day) for 10 days, then tapered over 3 weeks. Other dosage schedules were not investigated.

In Europe, pain associated with herpes zoster has been successfully treated with levodopa,[67] an anti-parkinsonian agent previously demonstrated effective in relieving the pain associated with bony metastases.[68-70] Five positive but uncontrolled reports were followed by an excellent double-blind study[67] of 47 out-patients randomly assigned to treatment with levodopa and benserazide (a peripheral decarboxylase inhibitor) or a lactose placebo. Patients received either levodopa 100 mg plus benserazide 25 mg or the placebo in capsular form orally three times daily for 10 days.

The placebo and levodopa groups were quite comparable in all regards, including average age (54 vs. 52 years), duration of lesions before treatment (2.9 vs. 3.1 days), and number of ''high risk'' patients, either older than 65 years or afflicted with ophthalmic zoster (9 vs. 10). Healing time for the cutaneous eruption averaged slightly greater than 2 weeks in both groups overall, but among high risk patients (including the elderly) average healing time was significantly reduced in the levodopa group (14 vs. 22 days). Average pain intensity was significantly less than controls in the high risk levodopa-treated patients after 2 days and after 3 days in the entire group. Overall postherpetic neuralgia was present after 60 days in 5 of 15 patients in the placebo group and only 1 of 16 patients in the levodopa group for whom complete data were available; these ratios were 4 of 7 and 1 of 8 in the high risk groups. While not statistically significant, these differences suggest that levodopa may reduce the incidence and/or duration of postherpetic neuralgia. Scarring of the skin was statistically less frequent among the high risk levodopa-treated patients. The only adverse effect of therapy was vomiting, which occurred in four patients with a mean age of 81 years (as well as in two young placebo-treated patients) and which the authors postulated could be avoided by initiating levodopa therapy at lower dosage.

More rapid healing and decreased pain during herpes zoster infection have also been reported for nonimmunocompromised patients treated with the guanine derivative acyclovir.[71] Consecutive patients hospitalized for herpes zoster were treated either with acyclovir 5 mg/kg or mannitol 100 mg (placebo) as an i.v. bolus every 8 hr for 5 days in a randomized double-blind trial. Using a somewhat complicated weighted clinical and photographic assessment, the 20 acyclovir-treated patients had statistically more rapid improvement than did the 22 controls. During the second week of the eruption, the proportion of patients in the acyclovir group reporting pain was statistically reduced by approximately half compared to that in the control group; this beneficial effect was more prominent for patients older than 67 years (approximately 10% in the acyclovir group vs. 65% in the control group) and for those beginning therapy within 3 days of the onset of symptoms. The authors do not state the overlap between these groups (the elderly and those seeking hospitalization within 3 days). Despite the initial differences, however, 1 and 3 months after discharge, there was no effect of treatment on the persistence of pain. No patient had adverse effects attributable to acyclovir. Improvements seen during the acute phase of the infection were attributed to the known antiviral effect of acyclovir.

Successful treatment of already established postherpetic neuralgia has been reported for both chlorprothixene[72] and a combination of psychtropic drugs,[73] although the anecdotal, unreported experience with these drugs has been disappointing. Patients with severe, long-standing neuralgia not responsive to the above measures should consult a center involved in the management of chronic pain, as less "conventional" approaches such as transcutaneous electrical stimulation may bring relief.

VI. BLISTERING DERMATOSES IN THE ELDERLY

For nondermatologists, blistering disorders of the skin frequently evoke confused and confusing differential diagnoses of entities they have rarely seen and possibly never managed. The list of disorders to be considered in older patients is not long, however, and can be conveniently subdivided into: (1) immunoglobulin-mediated diseases, (2) drug reactions, (3) bullae attributable to underlying metabolic disorders, and (4) bullae precipitated by direct physical trauma in anatomically predisposed skin. This discussion will concern the more common, better described blistering disorders of the elderly (Table 3); vesicular eruptions (e.g., herpes zoster), and the inflammatory dermatoses in which bullae may be a minor component (e.g., lupus erythematosus, lichen planus) are excluded.

Of the disorders listed, only bullous pemphigoid is strikingly more common in the elderly than in middle-aged adults. This seems at first anomalous, since like young children the elderly appear to have a lower threshold for experimental blister formation than young and middle-aged adults in response to standardized stimulae; yet young children frequently develop blisters in the course of certain infections and inflammatory disorders of the skin which do not cause blisters in adults. Perhaps the increased propensity for dermal-epidermal separation in the elderly (Chapter 3) is counterbalanced by muting of the inflammatory response (columns 1 and 2) or the failure of patients at high risk (columns 3 and 4) to survive into old age.

A. Bullous Pemphigoid
1. Clinical Features

Bullous pemphigoid (BP) is an idiopathic, immunoglobulin-mediated disease, first differentiated clinically and histologically from the much less common pemphigus vulgaris (PV) approximately 30 years ago.[74] Since then, it has been extensively studied and its pathogenesis is presently among the best understood of all dermatologic diseases,[75] although many questions remain. The elderly are affected most commonly,[76,77] and conversely, BP is almost certainly the most common blistering disease affecting older patients. Untreated, BP varies in severity from mild to disabling[78] and may be fatal. The disease is self-limited, lasting months to years,[79,80] with recurrences following disease-free periods in a substantial minority of patients.[81]

BP is characterized clinically by large, tense bullae arising on either erythematous or normal

Table 3
DIFFERENTIAL DIAGNOSIS FOR BLISTERING DERMATOSES IN THE ELDERLY

Immunoglobulin mediated diseases	Drug reactions	Bullae due to metabolic diseases	Bullae due to direct trauma
Bullous pemphigoid	Toxic epidermal necrolysis (TEN)	Bullosis diabeticorum	Ischemic blisters
Pemphigus vulgaris	Bullous drug eruption	Bullous dermatosis of hemodialysis (uremia)	Pressure (neuropathic)
	Contact dermatitis	Porphyria cutanea tarda	Edema/anasarca

appearing skin[82] (Plate 3).* Preceding or accompanying pruritus is common and may be intense.[82] Blisters occur most often on the trunk and proximal extremities. Approximately one-third of patients have oral lesions,[79,82] although unlike pemphigus vulgaris, the mouth is rarely the initial site of involvement. In some patients, bullae remain localized to one area for several months, and in a small group, the lesions never become widespread. Crusted erosions and urticarial wheals may coexist with intact bullae; hemorrhagic bullae are not unusual.

2. Diagnosis

The diagnosis of BP is confirmed by skin biopsy of an early lesion.[83] In most cases, routine sections stained with hematoxylin and eosin allow definitive diagnosis, although rarely the findings are also coexistent with dermatitis herpetiformis,[83] a disorder characterized clinically by intensely pruritic bilateral symmetric grouped vesicles and bullae. Immunofluorescent staining of perilesional skin is virtually pathognomonic in BP. Linear deposition of C_3 in all patients[84,85] and of IgG in most patients[86,87] occurs along the basement membrane zone (BMZ) and has been determined to be within the lamina lucida by immunoelectron microscopy.[88-90] Linear deposition of IgA or IgM in addition to C_3 and IgG is present in approximately 25%.[81,91] Indirect immunofluorescent studies utilizing patient serum and monkey esophagus or other cutaneous preparation demonstrate anti-BMZ antibodies of the IgG class in approximately two-thirds of patients,[79,81] and probably more often if the disease is widespread. The only other disorder with similar immunofluorescent findings, cicatricial pemphigoid,[78,80] is much less common and can readily be distinguished on clinical grounds. Hence, optimal initial evaluation of a patient with widespread BP includes a biopsy of one or more early lesions (or perilesional skin) for both routine histology and immunofluorescent studies, to be evaluated by an experienced dermatopathologist. A single 4-mm punch specimen may be bisected and each half processed separately. For the sake of economy and convenience, it may be preferable to request that immunofluorescent studies be performed only if diagnosis cannot be made on the basis of the histologic findings alone.

3. Treatment

Corticosteroids are the mainstay of therapy. In mild or localized cases, topical application of a potent steroid cream once or twice daily may control the lesions, but most patients require prednisone or its equivalent. Dosage and schedule of administration are determined by the extent, severity, and rate of progression of the disease as well as by patient age and the presence or absence of relative contraindications, such as hypertension, diabetes, osteoporosis, or infection.

Patients with extensive and/or rapidly progressive, disabling BP should begin therapy with

---

* Plate 3 appears after page 100.

prednisone 60 to 100 mg daily[78] (some authors recommend 2 to 3 times this dose[80]). They should be reevaluated at weekly intervals, and the prednisone reduced rapidly (e.g., 10 to 20 mg/week) as new blisters cease forming and clinical remission is achieved. An immunosuppressant such as daily azothioprine[93] 150 mg or cyclophosphamide 100 mg[94] may be added to the regimen initially or at the time of remission in order to reduce the eventual maintenance level of prednisone; 6 to 8 weeks are required for full expression of the steroid-sparing effect.

Patients with less severe BP may initiate therapy with alternate day prednisone 40 to 60 mg and/or daily use of an immunosuppressant. Drug dosages are decreased gradually to zero over many months, provided the disease remains in remission.

Sulfapyridine or sulfones[82,95] may be valuable alternative therapies for patients with major contraindications to systemic steroids. Most patients achieve prolonged remissions and at least half can ultimately discontinue treatment without recurrence of lesions.[96] Frequent exacerbation of the BP and potential complications of therapy require close monitoring of all patients throughout the course of their disease, however.

Concern that BP might be a marker for concurrent or subsequent development of malignancy[97] has not been substantiated by controlled studies.[80] The prevalence of malignant neoplasms appears to be approximately 10 to 11% in both patients with BP and their elderly, age-matched controls.[98,99]

B. Pemphigus Vulgaris

1. Clinical Features

Pemphigus vulgaris (PV, from the Greek, ''common blistering'') is a rare, autoimmune, immunoglobulin-mediated[100] disease of skin and mucous membranes which occurs predominantly in people of Jewish or Mediterranean ancestry.[74] Onset is most common in middle-age, although PV may first appear very late in life.[101] In contrast to BP, the untreated disease is relentlessly progressive and debilitating in most patients. PV was nearly universally fatal before the availability of corticosteroids and the mortality rate remains high due to the major adverse effects of prolonged high-dose systemic steroids necessary to control the disease in many patients.[102]

Mucous membranes, especially the buccal mucosae, are frequently involved and are the initial site of lesions in up to half of all patients.[102] The cervix, rectum, conjunctivae, and esophagus may also be involved. Intact blisters are uncommon; painful sometimes hemorrhagic erosions are the major manifestation. Cutaneous lesions include flaccid bullae, crusted or weeping erosions (Plate 4),* and in extensive or rapidly progressive cases a positive Nikolsky sign (dislodging of normal-appearing epidermis from the underlying dermis with lateral digital pressure, i.e., firm stroking of the skin). Lesions may remain confined to small areas for many weeks, but the course is generally one of progressive involvement, culminating in sepsis, debility, and death.

2. Diagnosis

The diagnosis of PV is confirmed by biopsy of an early lesion of the skin or mucous membrane. Routine histologic sections frequently demonstrate the pathognomonic suprabasilar cleft and loss of adhesion between keratinocytes which then float freely within the epidermal blister cavity (''acantholysis'')[82] and indeed may be detected by Tsanck preparations of material scraped from the floor of a blister cavity.[102] An infiltrate of eosinophils is frequently present and may precede the blister information.[103]

Direct immunofluorescent staining of lesional or perilesional skin is the most sensitive laboratory method for diagnosis of PV. In lesional skin, virtually all patients demonstrate

---

* Plate 4 appears after page 100.

uniform intercellular epidermal staining with C_3 and IgG directed against the glycocalyx of the "intercellular cement;"[80] at least 50% have identical C_3 deposition in uninvolved skin. Intercellular IgA and IgM deposition is also present in 25 to 40% of lesional or apparently normal skin.[101,104] Positive intercellular staining is present very early in the disease course and may persist for years after blister formation has been halted by treatment.[80]

Indirect immunofluorescent staining of an appropriate substratum such as monkey esophagus by patient serum frequently demonstrates patient antibodies directed against the intercellular substance, but may be negative early in the disease course, and is generally less a sensitive test for PV than direct immunofluorescence.[80]

3. Treatment

The principles of treatment closely parallel those discussed for BP, but the PV itself and the medications required for its control are most often life-threatening. Patients with extensive or rapidly progressive PV should be hospitalized and begun on high daily steroid doses (prednisone 180 to 360 mg or its equivalent) until new lesions cease and existing lesions heal.[80,102] Dosage increments of at least 60 mg daily are recommended at 5-day intervals until control is achieved. Inadequate initial steroid dosage is considered the most common cause of treatment failure and may complicate subsequent management of the patient. The anticipated toxicity of this regimen, which must be continued for at least 6 weeks in most patients, is obviously quite high in the elderly, and close monitoring is essential. Mortality attributable to this phase of therapy is approximately 10% even in unselected, predominantly middle-aged patient groups.[105]

As soon as the blistering is controlled, steroid dosage should be reduced as rapidly as possible, usually over several weeks, to an alternate day schedule of prednisone 40 mg. The patient's lesions and general well-being should be assessed clinically at weekly intervals during this time. Repeat determinations of serum antibody titers may also be used to assess disease control, although correlations of this titer with blistering activity is poor in some patients. An immunosuppressant (methotrexate, cyclophosphamide, or azothioprine) should be initiated as the steroid dosage is reduced in order to minimize the prednisone requirement.[80,102] Once the patient is controlled on alternate day prednisone, the dose should be slowly but progressively decreased until blistering resumes or the drug is eliminated. Patients usually require a year or more to successfully discontinue prednisone. In some patients, it is then possible to taper and discontinue the immunosuppressant over several months without reactivating the disease.

Patients diagnosed while the disease is still mild and limited in extent frequently enter remission following treatment with moderate daily or alternate daily prednisone dosage alone, or with an adjunctive immunosuppressant. In some patients an immunosuppressant alone may prevent progression of mild disease.[105-107] Chrysotherapy (intramuscular gold sodium thiomalate) has also been reported as a successful alternative or supplement for the above agents in patients with mild to moderate PV,[108] although it is anecdotally less effective than immunosuppressants in most patients.[80]

It is clear that the key to successful therapy of PV, especially in the elderly, is early diagnosis. This in turn requires a high index of suspicion and willingness to evaluate unexplained blisters or erosions.

C. Drug Reactions

In general, older patients are more sensitive to both the therapeutic and potential adverse effects of medications.[109] Age-related decreases in lean body mass, whole body water content, and renal function undoubtedly account for part of the sensitivity to medications such as penicillin, sulfonamides, tetracycline, and gold; alterations in drug absorption and metabolism may also be implicated.

Adverse drug reactions manifested in the skin occur in 2 to 4%[110,111] of hospitalized patients, with an average reaction rate per course of drug therapy of approximately 3 per 1000.[112] One in-patient survey involving more than 11,000 patients in nine hospitals revealed that 5.5% of all drug exposures resulted in an adverse reaction and that 28% of all patients (30 to 33% of the elderly) were affected. Hospitalization was either necessitated or strongly influenced by the drug reaction in 4% of patients. Drug rashes, some severe, accounted for 8.3% of the reactions overall.[112a] Exanthematous ("maculopapular") eruptions comprised nearly half of these cases and urticarial eruptions nearly one-fourth.[113]

From these data it is apparent that blistering drug reactions are uncommon. Nevertheless, bullous drug eruptions, erythema multiforme, fixed drug eruptions, drug-induced toxic epidermal necrolysis, and phototoxic reactions should be considered in elderly patients with blisters or erosions of uncertain etiology. Table 4 lists some of the more commonly used drugs implicated in these reactions. Statistically, allergic reactions are most likely to occur within the first week after initiating therapy,[114] but may begin at any time while on therapy and for at least 2 weeks after the last drug dose. Eruptions associated with sporadically used medications, self-prescribed OTC medications, or with agents such as food additives not regarded by the patient as drugs may be particularly difficult to diagnose.

D. Bullosis Diabeticorum

Unexplained blister formation by diabetic patients has been described for at least 50 years.[115,116] The bullae are characteristically painless, tense, noninflamed, and located on the lower extremities in ambulatory patients.[115-119] Lesions tend to arise suddenly and resolve slowly, sometimes with residual atrophy or scarring.[119] In many but not all reported patients the diabetes mellitus was long-standing, complicated by peripheral neuropathy, and poorly controlled at the time the lesions occurred.[119,120]

Histologically, the bullae are subepidermal with few inflammatory cells and no evidence of infection; the overlying epidermis lacks deep rete ridges and the walls of dermal venules are markedly thickened.[119]

The etiology of these blisters is conjectural, but is almost certainly related in part to repeated minor trauma of relatively insensitive skin.[119] Diabetic microangiopathy, as manifested by thickened dermal venules, may also be contributory.[119,121]

The absence of specific effective treatment, rational management consists of controlling the diabetes itself, and minimizing trauma to the involved sites. Individual bullae should not be opened, if possible, in order to avoid infection. Ruptured bullae should be managed as discussed in Section V.

E. Bullous Dermatosis of Hemodialysis (Uremia)

Blisters of unknown etiology have been reported in patients undergoing maintenance hemodialysis.[122-125] Up to 4% of patients with end stage renal disease may have a blistering eruption,[126] although the lesions are attributed to furosemide by some investigators[127,128] and definitely represent porphyria cutanea tarda (PCT) in some cases.[129-134] The "bullous dermatosis" is characterized by tense bullae, sometimes hemorrhagic, situated on the dorsa of the hands and other sun-exposed areas. Erosions may also be present, but milia and facial hypertrichosis (common features of PCT) have been absent in reported cases. A history relating lesions to sun exposure often cannot be elicited.

Histologically the lesion is a subepidermal bulla with minimal perivascular lymphocytic infiltration; the superficial dermis is edematous, with hypogranulated mast cells and markedly thickened venular walls.[122] Immunofluorescent studies reveal small, inconstant immunoglobulin deposits primarily in a perivenular distribution consistent with nonspecific vascular injury.[122] The clinical and histologic features of these bullae strongly suggest repeated low-grade phototoxic injury, similar to that in PCT, as the pathogenesis, although phototesting

Table 4

COMMON DRUGS OCCASIONALLY IMPLICATED AS CAUSES OF BLISTERING SKIN REACTIONS

Erythema multiforme	Fixed drug eruptions	Bullous drug eruptions
Barbiturates	Barbiturates	Barbiturates
Chlorpropamide	Estrogens/progestins	Halides
Griseofulvin	Meprobamate	Penicillin
Hydantoins	Phenacetin	
Penicillin	Phenolphthalein	
Phenothiazines	Phenylbutazone	
Sulfonamides	Salicylates	
Thiazides	Sulfonamides	
	Tetracycline	

Toxic epidermal necrolysis	Phototoxic reactions	
Allopurinol		
Barbiturates	Griseofulvin	
Hydantoins	Nalidixic acid	
Phenylbutazone	Phenothiazines	
Penicillin	Psoralens	
Sulfonamides	Sulfonamides	
Tetracycline	Sulfonylureas	

Modified from Wintroub, B. U., et al., *Dermatology in General Medicine*, Fitzpatrick, T. B., et al., Eds., McGraw-Hill, New York, 1979, 555.

has been negative.[122] An underlying uremic microangiopathy[134] may further reduce the threshold for blister formation in these patients.

Management consists of carefully excluding PCT[122,129] and drug-induced phototoxicity (potentially treatable causes), use of broad spectrum sunscreen or protective clothing and meticulous care of existing lesions to avoid infection.

F. Porphyria Cutanea Tarda

1. Clinical Features

Porphyria cutanea tarda (PCT) is a porphyrin-induced photosensitivity disorders characterized by small tense blisters, slow-healing erosions, milia (small epidermal cysts formed during healing), abnormal skin fragility, diffuse hyperpigmentation and occasionally hirsutism and sclerodermatous changes, all restricted to sun-exposed skin.[135] In most cases, involvement is most prominent on the dorsa of the hands. Lesions are usually more numerous and more severe during the summer, but patients rarely relate exacerbations to specific periods of sun exposure.   The classic patient is a middle-aged male alcoholic[136,137] in whom PCT is attributed to a combination of ethanol-induced increased porphyrin synthesis, hepatic insufficiency, and increased dietary iron absorption.[138] However, PCT may occur at any age, and has been increasingly recognized in two groups receiving estrogen therapy (also known to induce porphyrin synthesis[139]), postmenopausal women and elderly men with prostatic carcinoma.[140-142]

2. Diagnosis

Increased porphyrin levels are the sine qua non of PCT. Urinary uroporphyrin, especially isomer I, is markedly elevated in most patients, and urinary 7-carboxyl porphyrins moderately elevated.[143,144] This fact allows rapid confirmation of PCT by Wood's lamp illumination of an acidified urine specimen, in which excess porphyrins fluoresce coral red after absorbing Soret band (405 mm) energy.[135] Fecal porphyrins, especially isocoproporphyrin, are also elevated in PCT,[143] and plasma porphyrins are elevated more than 40-fold above controls on the average,[145] permitting diagnosis in oliguric patients. Quantitative urinary and fecal porphyrin levels are necessary to exclude the much less common disorder, variegate porphyrin, which produces identical cutaneous lesions.[135]

Biopsy of a skin blister reveals subepidermal bulla formation with minimal inflammatory response.[135] Slight nonspecific immunoglobulin and complement deposition at the dermo-epidermal junction and in perivascular areas can be detected by appropriate immunofluorescent staining,[135] but do not resemble the patterns seen in BP or DH.

3. Treatment

Alcohol, supplementary estrogens and excess dietary or therapeutic iron should be eliminated if possible because of their role in provoking or exacerbating PCT.[135] Avoidance of prolonged direct sun exposure is also helpful. Nonopaque sun screens are of no benefit, however, as they block only UV light, not the visible (blue) spectrum responsible for porphyric lesions.

Phlebotomy is indicated for most patients. Removal of 500 mℓ whole blood every 2 weeks until serum hemoglobin reaches 10 to 11 g/dℓ or serum iron reaches 50 to 60 μg/dℓ, a total of 1.5 to 12 ℓ, is recommended[146,147] but may need to be revised downward for elderly patients. Individuals with congestive heart failure, angina, borderline pulmonary function or other underlying disease require careful monitoring during this period of iatrogenic anemia. Chloroquine[148-150] and more recently plasmaphoresis[151] have been proposed as alternative therapies for patients in whom phlebotomy is contraindicated. Resolution of skin lesions and return of porphyrin levels to the normal range require many months, but once attained, remissions are usually long-lasting and may be permanent.[135]

G. Bullae Due to Direct Trauma

Dermo-epidermal separation may occur in skin with insufficient oxygen and nutrient exchange either acutely or chronically. Intrinsically inadequate arterial blood flow or externally applied pressure, exceeding that within the cutaneous vascular plexus, may be responsible for the tissue ischemia. The blisters may arise on normal appearing skin or within erythematous macules. Decubitus ulcers, discussed earlier in this chapter, occasionally begin in this way. A second example is "barbiturate blisters," subepidermal bullae appearing over weight-bearing areas such as the heels and shoulders in deeply comatose patients lying a few hours or less in a single position. These lesions classically observed in patients recovering from drug overdoses, were initially attributed to the ingested agent itself, but later recognized to result from prolonged local tissue ischemia experienced during coma.[152] Patients who are comatose following a cerebrovascular accident or even during prolonged general anesthesia, are also at risk, especially if tissue perfusion is poor under baseline conditions.

The relationship of lesions to external pressure is often obscured by the fact that such blisters may first appear hours to days after the ischemic episode at a time when the patient is again conscious or at least positioned differently (Plate 5).* Even more difficult to identify correctly are ischemic bullae arising in conscious patients with diminished cutaneous sensation for whom ischemia is not painful. Uremic or diabetic patients with peripheral neu-

---

* Plate 5 appears after page 100.

ropathy, for example, may develop such bullae as a result of ill-fitting shoes, prolonged sitting with crossed ankles, or any other minor trauma.

Dermal edema of any etiology exerts pressure on the dermo-epidermal junction and may cause separation even in the absence of ischemia. Bulla formation is more likely, or occurs with a lower threshold, however, in skin already compromised by ischemia, scarring, or even the physiologic changes associated with advanced age itself. Such bullae may occur on the legs of ambulatory patient with edema secondary to local venous stasis or systemic disease; they are commonly associated with infiltrated intravenous lines and other causes of severe localized edema in hospitalized patients.

Early, correct identification of bullae due to regional ischemia or edema is important because differential diagnosis often includes local or systemic infection, adverse drug reactions, contact dermatitis, metabolic abnormalities such as porphyria, and bullous pemphigoid. The diagnosis is supported by the absence of bacteria and inflammatory cells in blister aspirates. Skin biopsy is often contraindicated by the lesion's location and clinical setting; histologic findings vary with etiology and duration of the blister but frequently do permit exclusion of alternative etiologies when diagnosis cannot be made on clinical grounds alone.

There is no specific therapy for these bullae and none is necessary. Once the underlying ischemia or edema is corrected, healing occurs either through re-epithelialization or resorption of the blister fluid with re-attachment at the dermo-epidermal junction.

REFERENCES

1. **Agris, J. and Spira, M.,** Pressure ulcers: prevention and treatment, *Ciba Clin. Symposia*, 31, 1979.
2. **Bennett, L., Kavner, D., Lee, B. Y., Trainor, F. S., and Lewis, J. M.,** Skin blood flow in seated geriatric patients, *Arch. Phys. Med. Rehabil.*, 62, 392, 1981.
3. **Kligman, A. M.,** Perspectives and problems in cutaneous gerontology, *J. Invest. Dermatol.*, 73, 39, 1979.
4. **Pearce, R. H. and Grimmer, B. J.,** Age and the chemical constitution of normal human dermis, *J. Invest. Dermatol.*, 58, 347, 1972.
5. **Johnson, M. L. T. and Roberts, J.,** Prevalence of dermatological disease among persons 1—74 years of age: United States, Advance Data No. 4, USHDEW, 1977.
6. **Tonnesen, M. G.,** Pruritus, in *Dermatology in General Medicine*, 2nd ed., Fitzpatrick, T. B., Eisen, A. Z., Wolff, K., et al., Eds., McGraw-Hill, New York, 1979, 32.
7. **Lyell, A.,** The itching patient: a review of the causes of pruritus, *Scott. Med. J.*, 17, 324, 1972.
8. **Beare, J. M.,** Generalized pruritus: a study of 43 cases, *Clin. Exp. Dermatol.*, 17, 334, 1876.
9. **Gilchrest, B. A., Stoff, J. S., and Soter, N. A.,** Chronologic aging alters the response to UV-induced inflammation of human skin, *J. Invest. Dermatol.*, 79, 11, 1982.
10. **Fitzpatrick, T. B., Eisen, A. Z., Wolff, K., et al.,** *Dermatology in General Medicine*, McGraw-Hill, New York, 1978.
11. **Rajka, G.,** Investigation of patients suffering from generalized pruritus with special reference to systemic diseases, *Acta Derm. Venereol.*, 49, 190, 1966.
12. **Botero, F.,** Pruritus as a manifestation of systemic disorders, *Cutis*, 21, 873, 1978.
13. **Makipour, H., Cooperman, A., Danzi, J. T., et al.,** Carcinoma of the ampulla of Vater: review of 38 cases with emphasis on treatment and prognostic factors, *Ann. Surg.*, 183, 341, 1976.
14. **Thorne, E. G.,** Coping with pruritus: a common geriatric complaint, *Geriatrics*, 33, 47, 1978.
15. **Easton, P. and Gailbraith, P. R.,** Cimetidine treatment of pruritus in polycythemia vera, *N. Engl. J. Med.*, 229, 1134, 1978.
16. **Klein, H.,** *Polycythemia: Theory and Management*, Charles C Thomas, Springfield, Ill., 1973, 96.
17. **Winkelman, R. K.,** Dermatologic clinics. I. Comments on pruritus related to systemic disease, *Proc. Staff Meetings Mayo Clin.*, 36, 187, 1961.
18. **Bluefarb, S. M.,** *Cutaneous Manifestations of Malignant Lymphomas*, Charles C Thomas, Springfield, Ill., 1959, 534.

19. **Feuner, A. S., Mahmood, T., and Willner, S. F.,** Prognostic importance of pruritus in Hodgkin's disease, *JAMA,* 240, 2738, 1978.
20. **Lamberg, S. I., Green, S. B., Byar, D. P., et al.,** Status report of 376 mycosis fungoides patients at four years. Mycosis Fungoides Cooperative Group, *Cancer Treat. Rep.,* 63, 701, 1979.
21. **Erskine, J. G., Rowan, R. M., Alexander, J. O., et al.,** Pruritus as a presentation of myelomatosis, *Br. J. Med.,* 1, 687, 1977.
22. **Zelicovici, A.,** Pruritus as a possible early sign of paraproteinemia, *Isr. J. Med. Sci.,* 5, 1079, 1969.
23. **Lewiecki, E. M. and Rahman, F.,** Pruritus: a manifestation of iron deficiency, *JAMA,* 236, 2319, 1976.
24. **Vickers, C. F.,** Iron-deficiency pruritus, *JAMA,* 238, 129, 1977.
25. **Barnes, H. M., Sarkany, I., and Calnan, C. D.,** Pruritus and thyrotoxicosis, *Trans. St. Johns Hosp. Dermatol. Soc.,* 60, 59, 1974.
26. **Besdine, R. W.,** Geriatric medicine: an overview, in *Annual Review of Gerontology and Geriatrics,* Eisdorfer, C., Ed., Springer Publishing Co., New York, 1980, 145.
27. **Greenwood, A. M.,** A study of the skin in 500 cases of diabetes, *JAMA,* 89, 774, 1927.
28. **Stawiski, M. A. and Voorhees, J. J.,** Cutaneous signs of diabetes mellitus, *Cutis,* 18, 415, 1976.
29. **Cornia, F. E.,** Pruritus, an uncommon but important symptom of systemic carcinoma, *Arch. Dermatol.,* 92, 36, 1965.
30. **Rothman, S.,** Physiology of itching, *Physiol. Rev.,* 21, 357, 1941.
31. **Felding, W. and Paton, W. D. M.,** Release of histamine from skin and muscle in the cat by opium alkaloids and other histamine liberators, *J. Physiol.,* 114, 490, 1951.
32. **Griesmer, R. D. and Nadelson, T.,** Emotional aspects of cutaneous disease, in *Dermatology in General Medicine,* 2nd ed., Fitzpatrick, T. B., Eisen, A. Z., Wolff, K., et al., Eds., McGraw-Hill, New York, 1979, 1353.
33. **Hobson, W. and Pemberton, J.,** *The Health of the Elderly at Home,* Butterworths, London, 1955, 53.
34. **Gilchrest, B. A.,** Pruritus: pathogenesis, therapy and significance in systemic disease states, *Arch. Intern. Med.,* 142, 101, 1982.
35. **Massry, S. G., Popovtzer, M. M., Coburn, J. W., et al.,** Intractable pruritus as a manifestation of secondary hyperparathyroidism in uremia, *N. Engl. J. Med.,* 279, 697, 1968.
36. **Hampers, C. L., Katz, A. I., and Wilson, R. E.,** Disappearance of "uremic" itching after subtotal parathyroidectomy, *N. Engl. J. Med.,* 279, 695, 1968.
37. **Tapia, L., Cheigh, J. S., David, D. S., et al.,** Pruritus in dialysis patients treated with parenteral lidocaine, *N. Engl. J. Med.,* 296, 261, 1977.
38. **Gilchrest, B. A., Rowe, J. W., Brown, R. S., et al.,** Ultraviolet phototherapy of uremic pruritus: long term results and possible mechanisms of action, *Ann. Intern. Med.,* 91, 17, 1979.
39. **Shultz, B. C. and Roenigk, H. H., Jr.,** Uremic pruritus treated with ultraviolet light, *JAMA,* 243, 1836, 1980.
40. **Silverberg, D. S., Iaina, A., Reisin, E., et al.,** Cholestyramine in uremic pruritus, *Br. Med. J.,* 1, 752, 1977.
41. **Pederson, J. A., Matter, B. J., Czerwinski, A. W., et al.,** Relief of idiopathic generalized pruritus in dialysis patients treated with activated oral charcoal, *Ann. Intern. Med.,* 93, 446, 1980.
42. **Corey, J. B. and Williams, G.,** Relief of the pruritus of jaundice with a bile acid sequestering resin, *JAMA,* 176, 432, 1961.
43. **Lottsfeldt, F. I., Krwit, W., Anst, J. B., et al.,** Cholestyramine therapy in intrahepatic biliary atresia, *N. Engl. J. Med.,* 269, 186, 1963.
44. **Rosenoer, V. M. and Gokin, G., Jr.,** Management of patients with chronic obstructive jaundice, *Med. Clin. North Am.,* 56, 759, 1972.
45. **Lauterburg, B. H., Pineda, A. A., Dickson, E. R., et al.,** Plasma perfusion for the treatment of intractable pruritus of cholestasis, *Mayo Clin. Proc.,* 53, 403, 1978.
46. **Arndt, K. A.,** *Manual of Dermatologic Therapeutics,* 2nd ed., Little, Brown, Boston, 1978, 263.
47. **Zappacosta, A. R. and Haus, D.,** Cimetidine doesn't help pruritus of uremia, *N. Engl. J. Med.,* 300, 1280, 1979.
48. **Vestal, R. E.,** Drug use in the elderly: a review of problems and special considerations, *Drugs,* 16, 358, 1978.
49. **Oxman, M. N.,** Varicella and herpes zoster, in *Dermatology in General Medicine,* Fitzpatrick, T. B., Eisen, A. Z., Wolff, K., Freedberg, I. M., and Austen, K. F., Eds., McGraw-Hill, New York, 1979, 1600.
50. **Hope-Simpson, R. E.,** The nature of herpes zoster: a long-term study and a new hypothesis, *Proc. R. Soc. Med.,* 58, 9, 1965.
51. **Bourgoon, C. F., Burgoon, J. S., and Baldridge, G. D.,** The natural history of herpes zoster, *JAMA,* 164, 265, 1957.

52. **deMoragas, J. M. and Kierland, R. R.,** The outcome of patients with herpes zoster, *Arch. Dermatol.,* 75, 193, 1957.

53. **Oberg, G. and Svedmyr, A.,** Varicelliform eruptions in herpes zoster — some clinical and serological observations, *Scand. J. Infect. Dis.,* 1, 47, 1969.

54. **Shanbrom, E., et al.,** Herpes zoster in hematologic neoplasias: some unusual manifestations, *Ann. Intern. Med.,* 53, 523, 1960.

55. **Sokal, J. E. and Firat, D.,** Varicella-zoster infection in Hodgkin's disease, *Am. J. Med.,* 39, 452, 1965.

56. **Schimpff, S., et al.,** Varicella-zoster infection in patients with cancer, *Ann. Intern. Med.,* 76, 241, 1972.

57. **Goffinet, D. R., et al.,** Herpes zoster-varicella infections and lymphoma, *Ann. Intern. Med.,* 76, 235, 1972.

58. **Juel-Jensen, B. E. and Maccallum, F. O.,** *Herpes Simplex, Varicella and Zoster,* Lippincott, Philadelphia, 1972.

59. **Easton, H. G.,** Zoster sine herpete causing trigeminal neuralgia, *Lancet,* 2, 1065, 1970.

60. **Luby, J. P., et al.,** A longtitudinal study of varicella-zoster virus infections in renal transplant recipients, *J. Infect. Dis.,* 135, 659, 1977.

61. **Barr, R. J., et al.,** Rapid method for Tzanck preparations, *JAMA,* 237, 1119, 1977.

62. **Bruusgaard, E.,** The mutual relation between zoster and varicella, *Br. J. Dermatol. Syphilol.,* 44, 1, 1932.

63. **Ragozzino, M. W., Melton, L. J., Kurland, L. T., Chu, C. P., and Perry, H. O.,** Risk of cancer after herpes zoster: a population-based study, *N. Engl. J. Med.,* 307, 393, 1982.

64. **Sultzberger, M. B., Sauter, G. C., Herrmann, F., Baer, R. L., and Milberg, I. L.,** Effects of ACTH and cortisone on certain diseases and physiological functions of the skin. I. Effects of ACTH, *J. Invest. Dermatol.,* 16, 323, 1951.

65. **Eaglstein, W. H., Katz, R., and Brown, J. A.,** The effects of corticosteroid therapy on the skin eruption and pain of herpes zoster, *JAMA,* 211, 1681, 1970.

66. **Keczkes, K. and Basheer, A. M.,** Do corticosteroids prevent post-herpetic neuralgia? *Br. J. Dermatol.,* 102, 551, 1980.

67. **Kernbaum, S. and Hauchecorne, J.,** Administration of Levodopa for relief of herpes zoster pain, *JAMA,* 246, 132, 1981.

68. **Dickey, R. and Minton, J.,** Levodopa relief of bone pain from breast cancer, *N. Engl. J. Med.,* 286, 843, 1972.

69. **Minton, J.,** The response of breast cancer patients with bone pain to l-dopa, *Cancer,* 33, 358, 1974.

70. **Nixon, D.,** Use of l-dopa to relieve pain from bone metastases, *N. Engl. J. Med.,* 292, 647, 1975.

71. **Peterslund, N. A., Ipsen, J., Schonheyder, H., Seyer-Hansen, K., Esmann, V., and Juhl, H.,** Acyclovir in herpes zoster, *Lancet,* 2, 827, 1981.

72. **Kramer, P. W.,** The management of post herpetic neuralgia with chlorprothixene, *Surg. Neurol.,* 15, 102, 1981.

73. **Taub, A.,** Relief of postherpetic neuralgia with psychotropic drugs, *J. Neurosurg.,* 39, 235, 1973.

74. **Lever, W. F.,** Pemphigus, *Medicine (Baltimore),* 32, 1, 1953.

75. **Sams, W. M., Jr. and Gammon, W. R.,** Mechanism of lesions production in pemphigus and pemphigoid, *J. Am. Acad. Dermatol.,* 6, 431, 1982.

76. **Rook, A. and Waddinton, E.,** Pemphigus and pemphoid, *Br. J. Dermatol.,* 65, 425, 1953.

77. **Sneddon, I. B. and Church, R.,** Diagnosis and treatment of pemphigoid: report on 22 cases, *Br. Med. J.,* 2, 1360, 1955.

78. **Jordon, R. E.,** Bullous pemphigoid, cicatricial pemphigoid, and chronic bullous dermatosis of childhood, in *Dermatology in General Medicine,* Fitzpatrick, T. B., Eisen, A. Z., Wolff, K., Freedberg, I. M., and Austen, K. F., Eds., McGraw-Hill, New York, 1979, 318.

79. **Person, J. R. and Rogers, R. S., III,** Bullous and cicatricial pemphigoid. Clinical, histopathologic and immunopathologic correlations, *Mayo Clin. Proc.,* 52, 54, 1977.

80. **Lever, W. F.,** Pemphigus and pemphigoid, *J. Am. Acad. Dermatol.,* 1, 2, 1979.

81. **Ahmed, A. R., Maize, J. C., and Provost, T. T.,** Bullous pemphigoid. Clinical and immunologic follow-up after successful therapy, *Arch. Dermatol.,* 112, 185, 1977.

82. **Lever, W. F.,** *Pemphigus and Bullous Pemphigoid,* Charles C Thomas, Springfield, Ill. 1965, 222.

83. **Eng, A. M. and Moncada, B.,** Bullous pemphigoid and dermatitis herpetiformis. Histopathologic differentiation of bullous pemphigoid and dermatitis herpetiformis, *Arch. Dermatol.,* 110, 51, 1978.

84. **Chorzelski, T. P. and Cormane, R. H.,** The presence of complement bound in vivo in the skin of patients with pemphigoid, *Dermatologica,* 137, 134, 1968.

85. **Provost, T. T. and Tomasi, T. B., Jr.,** Immunopathology of bullous pemphigoid: basement membrane deposition of IgE, alternate pathway components and fibrin, *Clin. Exp. Immunol.,* 18, 193, 1974.

86. **Jordon, R. E., Beutner, E. H., and Witebsky, E.,** Basement zone antibodies in bullous pemphigoid, *JAMA,* 200, 751, 1967.

87. **Chorzelski, T., Jablonska, S., Blaszczyk, M., and Zarzabek, M.,** Autoantibodies in pemphigoid, *Dermatologica,* 136, 325, 1968.
88. **Schmidt-Ullrich, B., Rule, A., Schaumburg-Lever, G., and Leblanc, S.,** Ultrastructural localization in vivo bound complement in bullous pemphigoid, *J. Invest. Dermatol.,* 65, 217, 1975.
89. **Holubar, K., Wolff, K., Konrad, K., and Beutner, E. H.,** Ultrastructural localization of immunoglobulins in bullous pemphigoid skin, *J. Invest. Dermatol.,* 64, 220, 1975.
90. **Wolff-Schreiner, E. and Wolff, K.,** Immunoglobulins at the dermal-epidermal junction in lupus erythematosus: ultrastructural investigation, *Arch. Dermatol. Res.,* 246, 193, 1973.
91. **Provost, T. T. and Tomasi, T. B., Jr.,** Immunopathology of bullous pemphigoid, *Clin. Exp. Immunol.,* 18, 193, 1974.
92. **Tuffanelli, D. L.,** Cutaneous immunopathology: recent observations, *J. Invest. Dermatol.,* 65, 143, 1975.
93. **Burton, J. L. and Greaves, M. W.,** Azathioprine for pemphigus and pemphigoid: a four year study follow-up, *Br. J. Dermatol.,* 91, 103, 1974.
94. **Krain, L. S.,** Cyclophosphamide in the treatment of pemphigus vulgaris and bullous pemphigoid, *Arch. Dermatol.,* 106, 657, 1972.
95. **Person, J. R. and Rogers, R. S., III,** Bullous pemphigoid responding to sulfapyridine and the sulfones, *Arch. Dermatol.,* 113, 610, 1977.
96. **Stevenson, C. J.,** Treatment in bullous disease with corticosteroid drugs and corticotrophin, *Br. J. Dermatol.,* 72, 11, 1960.
97. **Chorzelski, T. P., Jablonska, S., and Maciejowska, E.,** Coexistence of malignancies with bullous pemphigoid, *Arch. Dermatol.,* 114, 964, 1978.
98. **Lim, C. C., Macdonald, R. H., and Rook, A. J.,** Pemphigoid eruptions in the elderly, *Trans. St. John's Hosp. Dermatol. Soc.,* 54, 148, 1968.
99. **Stone, S. P. and Schroeter, A. L.,** Bullous pemphigoid and associated malignant neoplasms, *Arch. Dermatol.,* 11, 991, 1975.
100. **Anhalt, G. J., Labib, R. S., Voorhees, J. J., Beals, T. F., and Diaz, L. A.,** Induction of pemphigus in neonatal mice by passive transfer of IgG from patients with the disease, *N. Engl. J. Med.,* 306, 1189, 1982.
101. **Meurer, M.,** Oral pemphigus vulgaris: a report of 10 cases, *Arch. Dermatol.,* 113, 1520, 1977.
102. **Jordon, R. E.,** Pemphigus, in *Dermatology in General Medicine,* Fitzpatrick, T. B., Eisen, A. Z., Wolff, K., Freedberg, I. M., and Austen, K. F., Eds., McGraw-Hill, New York, 1979, 310.
103. **Emmerson, R. W. and Wilson, J. E.,** Eosinophilic spongiosis in pemphigus: a report of an unusual histological change in pemphigus, *Arch. Dermatol.,* 97, 252, 1968.
104. **Judd, K. P. and Lever, W. F.,** Correlations of antibodies in skin and serum with disease severity in pemphigus, *Arch. Dermatol.,* 115, 428, 1979.
105. **Lever, W. F. and Schaumburg-Lever, G.,** Immunosuppressants and prednisone in pemphigus vulgaris. Therapeutic results obtained in 63 patients between 1961 and 1975, *Arch. Dermatol.,* 113, 1236, 1977.
106. **Roenigk, H. H., Jr. and Doedhar, S.,** Pemphigus treated with azathioprine *Arch. Dermatol.,* 107, 353, 1973.
107. **Van Dijk, T. J. A. and van Velde, J. L.,** Treatment of pemphigus and pemphigoid with azathioprine, *Dermatologica,* 147, 179, 1973.
108. **Penneys, N. S., Eaglstein, W. H., and Frost, P.,** Management of pemphigus with gold compounds: a long-term follow-up report, *Arch. Dermatol.,* 112, 185, 1976.
109. **Vestal, R. E.,** Drug use in the elderly: a review of problems and special considerations, *Drugs,* 16, 358, 1978.
110. **Shapiro, S., Slone, D., Siskind, V., et al.,** Drug rash with ampicillin and other penicillins, *Lancet,* 2, 969, 1969.
111. **Jick, H., Miettinen, O. S., Shapiro, S., et al.,** Comprehensive drug surveillance, *JAMA,* 213, 1455, 1970.
112. **Arndt, K. A. and Jick, H.,** Rates of cutaneous reactions to drugs: a report from the Boston Collaborative Drug Surveillance Program, *JAMA,* 235, 918, 1976.
112a. **Miller, R. R.,** Drug surveillance utilizing epidemiologic methods, *Am. J. Hosp. Pharm.,* 30, 584, 1973.
113. **Kuokkanen, L.,** Drug eruptions: a series of 464 cases in the Department of Dermatology, University of Turku, Finland, during 1966—1970, *Acta Allergol.,* 27, 407, 1972.
114. **Wintroub, B. U., Shiffman, N. J., and Arndt, K. A.,** Adverse cutaneous reactions to drugs, in *Dermatology in General Medicine,* Fitzpatrick, T. B., Eisen, A. Z., Wolff, K., Freedberg, I.M., and Austen, K. F., Eds., McGraw-Hill, New York, 1979, 555.
115. **Kramer, D. W.,** Early warning signs of impending gangrene in diabetes, *Med. J. Rec.,* 652, 338, 1930.
116. **Cope, R. L.,** Spontaneous bulla formation in the skin in diabetes mellitus, *Ann. Intern. Med.,* 32, 964, 1950.
117. **Rocca, R. P. and Pereyra, E.,** Phlyctenar lesions in the feet of diabetic patients, *Diabetes,* 12, 220, 1963.

118. **Cantwell, A. R. and Martz, W.**, Idiopathic bullae in diabetics, *Arch. Dermatol.*, 96, 42, 1967.
119. **Kurwa, A., Roberts, P., and Whitehead, R.**, Concurrence of bullous and atrophic skin lesions in diabetes mellitus, *Arch. Dermatol.*, 103, 670, 1971.
120. **Allen G. E. and Hadden, D. R.**, Bullous lesions of the skin in diabetes, *Br. J. Dermatol.*, 82, 216, 1970.
121. **Freinkel, R. K. and Freinkel, N.**, Dermatologic manifestations of endocrine disorders, in *Dermatology in General Medicine*, Fitzpatrick, T. B. et al., Eds., McGraw-Hill, New York, 1979, 1261.
122. **Gilchrest, B., Rowe, J. W., and Mihm, M. C.**, Bullous dermatosis of hemodialysis, *Ann. Intern. Med.*, 83, 480, 1975.
123. **Brivet, F., Drueke, T., Guillemette, J., et al.**, Porphyria cutanea tarda-like syndrome in hemodialyzed patients, *Nephron.*, 20, 258, 1978.
124. **Webster, S. B. and Dahlberg, P. J.**, Bullous dermatosis of hemodialysis, *Cutis,* 25, 322, 1980.
125. **Rothstein, H.**, Photosensitive bullous eruption associated with chronic renal failure, *Aust. J. Dermatol.*, 19, 58, 1979.
126. **Dymock, R. D.**, Skin diseases associated with renal transplantation, *Aust. J. Dermatol.*, 20, 61, 1979.
127. **Keczkes, K. and Farr, M.**, Bullous dermatosis of chronic renal failure, *Br. J. Dermatol.*, 95, 541, 1976.
128. **Burry, J. N. and Lawrence, J. R.**, Phototoxic blisters from high furosemide dosage, *Br. J. Dermatol.*, 94, 495, 1976.
129. **Poh-Fitzpatrick, M. B., Bettet, N., and DeLeo, V. A.**, Porphyria cutanea tarda in two patients treated with hemodialysis for chronic renal failure, *N. Engl. J. Med.*, 279, 292, 1978.
130. **Wilken, J. K., Kaplan, R. J., and Acchiardo, S. R.**, Porphyria cutanea tarda in a chronic hemodialysis patient, *South. Med. J.*, 73, 106, 1980.
131. **Topi, G. C., E'Alessandro, G. L., Cancarini, G. C., et al.**, Porphyria cutanea tarda in a hemodialyzed patient, *Br. J. Dermatol.*, 104, 579, 1981.
132. **Lichtenstein, J. R., Babb, E. J., and Felsher, B. F.**, Porphyria cutanea tarda (PCT) in a patient with chronic renal failure on hemodialysis, *Br. J. Dermatol.*, 104, 575, 1981.
133. **Parilla, J. G., Ortega, R., Pena, M. L., et al.**, Porphyria cutanea tarda during maintenance hemodialysis, *Br. Med. J.*, 1358, 1980.
134. **Hanno, R. and Callen, J. P.**, Porphyria cutanea tarda as a cause of bullous dermatosis of hemodialysis: a case report and review of the literature, *Cutis,* 28, 261, 1981.
135. **Bickers, D. R., Pathak, M. A., and Magnus, I. A.**, The porphyrias, in *Dermatology in General Medicine*, Fitzpatrick, T. B., Eisen, A. Z., Wolff, K., Freedberg, I. M., and Austen, K. F., Eds., McGraw-Hill, New York, 1979, 1072.
136. **Brunsting, L. A.**, Observations on porphyria cutanea tarda, *Arch. Dermatol. Syphilol.*, 70, 551, 1954.
137. **Stanley, B. C.**, Effect of ethanol on liver δ-aminolaevulinate synthetase activity and urinary porphyrin excretion in symptomatic porphyria, *Br. J. Haematol.*, 17, 389, 1969.
138. **Hourihane, D. O. and Webb, D. G.**, Suppression of erythropoiesis by alcohol, *Br. Med. J.*, 1, 86, 1970.
139. **Levere, R. D.**, Stilbesterol-induced porphyria: increase in hepatic δ-aminole-vulinic acid synthesis, *Blood*, 28, 569, 1966.
140. **Roenigk, H. H., Jr. and Gottlob, N. E.**, Estrogen-induced porphyria cutanea tarda, *Arch. Dermatol.*, 102, 260, 1970.
141. **Harber, L. C. and Bickers, D. R.**, The porphyrias: basic science aspects, clinical diagnosis, and management, in *Yearbook of Dermatology*, Malkinson, F. and Pearson, R., Eds., Year Book, Chicago, 1975, 9.
142. **Taylor, J. S. and Roenigk, H. H., Jr.**, Estrogen-induced porphyria cutanea tarda, in *Porphyrins in Human Disease*, Doss, M. and Marocki, P., Karger, Basel, 1976, 328.
143. **Elder, G. H.**, Porphyrin metabolism in porphyria cutanea tarda, *Semin. Hematol.*, 14, 227, 1977.
144. **Smith, S. G.**, Porphyrins found in urine of patient with symptomatic porphyria, *Biochem. Soc. Trans.*, 5, 1472, 1977.
145. **Poh-Fitzpatrick, M. B., Sosin, A. E., and Bemis, J.**, Porphyrin levels in plasma and erythrocytes of chronic hemodialysis patients, *J. Am. Acad. Dermatol.*, 7, 100, 1982.
146. **Epstein, J. H. and Redeker, A. G.**, Porphyria cutaea tarda: a study of the effect of phlebotomy, *N. Engl. J. Med.*, 279, 1301, 1968.
147. **Ramsay, C. A.**, The treatment of porphyria cutanea tarda by venesection, *Q. J. Med.*, 43, 1, 1974.
148. **Saltzer, E. I.**, Porphyria cutanea tarda: remission following chloroquine administration without adverse effects, *Arch. Dermatol.*, 98, 496, 1968.
149. **Kordac, V.**, Chloroquine in the treatment of porphyria cutanea tarda, *N. Engl. J. Med.*, 296, 949, 1977.
150. **Swanbeck, G. and Wennersten, G.**, Treatment of porphyria cutanea tarda with chloroquine and phlebotomy, *Br. J. Dermatol.*, 97, 77, 1977.
151. **Disler, P., Day, R., Burman, N., Blekkenhorst, G., and Eales, L.**, Treatment of hemodialysis-related porphyria cutanea tarda with plasma exchange, *Am. J. Med.*, 72, 989, 1982.
152. **Arndt, K. A., Mihm, M. C., Jr., and Parrish, J. A.**, Bullae: a cutaneous sign of a variety of neurological diseases, *J. Invest. Dermatol.*, 60, 312, 1973.

Chapter 5

PREMATURE AGING SYNDROMES AFFECTING THE SKIN

I. INTRODUCTION

In order to understand normal aging, medical scientists have sought to identify human diseases characterized by abnormal aging, an approach which has proven fruitful in the study of other physiologic processes. To date, no disease has been found to manifest a truly altered rate of aging[1] but there are several "premature aging syndromes," so categorized originally because of a wizened or aged overall appearance. Patients with these diseases do manifest certain features of advanced age in childhood or early adulthood, although discrepancies with normal aging are readily apparent.

George Martin, one of the country's foremost gerontologists, has reviewed all the recognized genetic diseases of man and from a list of 2300 entities has selected 162 "segmental progeroid syndromes," diseases with premature or accelerated development of certain clinical features associated with normal aging.[1] None of these syndromes has been thoroughly investigated from the dermatologic point of view to see if the skin actually meets stringent criteria for true premature or accelerated aging.[2-4] Nevertheless, these diseases often have striking cutaneous manifestations (Table 1).

Table 2 lists the disorders most frequently cited as exhibiting precocious or accelerated aging. Seven appear to be inherited in an autosomal recessive manner and are rare. Diabetes mellitus with its as yet undefined inheritance pattern and trisomy of chromosome 21 (Down's syndrome) are much more common. Although all the premature aging syndromes are congenital in the sense of harboring an inborn genetic defect, many are without clinical manifestations during the first months or years of life.

II. WERNER SYNDROME

In his 1904 doctoral dissertation entitled "Cataract in Combination with Scleroderma," the German ophthalmologist Werner described four siblings, two men and two women, aged 31 to 40 years, living in a remote rural valley region characterized by extensive inbreeding over many generations.[5] The patients had short stature and a "senile appearance," uniformly grey hair after age 30 years, subcapsular cataracts which matured rapidly in the third decade, joint contractures, early menopause, and debilitating skin changes. Later reports[6,7] added baldness, laryngeal atrophy with high-pitched voice, osteoporosis, clinical hypogonadism with probably reduced fertility, vascular calcification of the Monkeburg type, an increased risk of malignancy, and decreased life span to the syndrome. In at least some instances, patients with Werner syndrome clearly have mild growth failure even during the first decade of life, although correct diagnosis is possible only after other disease manifestations develop.[61] Intelligence appears to be within normal limits in all patients; a single case report mentions "senile dementia."[8] Death usually occurs in the fourth to sixth decade, due to myocardial infarction or metastatic malignancy.

Skin changes described in Werner syndrome include tautness, sclerosis, atrophy, hyperkeratosis, loss of subcutaneous fat, and chronic ulcerations not readily attributable to ischemia (Plate 6)*[7,9] Changes are most striking on the distal limbs, especially the feet, with relative sparing of the trunk. Successive amputations are often necessitated by nonhealing painful ulcers and/or acral gangrene. The face is "pinched," usually suggesting an individual 30 to 40 years older than the chronologic age. Skin cancers have been reported, although the incidence is not as striking as that of other malignancies, especially fibrosarcomas,[7,10] which

---

* Plate 6 appears after page 100.

Table 1
FEATURES OF PROGEROID
SYNDROMES SUGGESTED TO
REPRESENT PREMATURE AGING
OF THE SKIN AND ITS
APPENDAGES

Atrophy[a]	Hair loss
Greying of the hair (canities)	Poikiloderma
Persistent ulceration	Sclerosis
Pigmentary disturbance	Wrinkling
Loss of subcutaneous fat	Nail dystrophy

[a]   Term used to imply loss of dermal thickness with consequently prominent veins.

From Gilchrest, B. A., Premature aging syndromes affecting the skin, in *Morphogenesis and Malformation of the Skin,* Blandau, R. J., Ed., Alan R. Liss for the March of Dimes Birth Defects Foundation, New York, 1981, 227. With permission.

Table 2
DISORDERS FREQUENTLY CLASSIFIED AS
PREMATURE AGING SYNDROMES

Progeria	Werner syndrome	Generalized lipodystrophy
Acrogeria	Rothmund syndrome	Trisomy 21 (Down syndrome)
Metageria	Cockayne syndrome	Diabetes mellitus

From Gilchrest, B.A., Premature aging syndromes affecting the skin, in *Morphogenesis and Malformation of the Skin,* Blandau, R. J., Ed., Alan R. Liss for the March of Dimes Birth Defects Foundation, 1981, 227. With permission.

occur in approximately 10% of patients.[10] Of the approximately 150 reported cases of Werner syndrome, 1 had a malignant melanoma,[10] and at least 5 developed basal cell carcinomas of sun-exposed areas by the sixth decade.[9,11,12]

In the only reported histologic and biochemical studies of the skin in Werner syndrome, Fleischmajer and Nedwich,[8] analyzing a sclerodermatous area from the dorsum of an amputated foot, found (1) replacement of subcutaneous fat by hyalinized collagen, (2) increased amounts of hexosamine, hydroxyproline, and dermatan sulfate, probably attributable to the increased ratio of collagen to fat, and (3) vessel wall changes in the papillary dermis similar to those commonly seen in patients with diabetes mellitus.

In their classic article in 1966, Epstein et al. reviewed the 125 well-documented cases of Werner syndrome reported up to that time.[7] Their data strongly support an autosomal recessive inheritance with a calculated gene frequency of 1 to 5 per 1000 population. Etiology is unknown; postulated disorders of the thyroid, adrenal, and pituitary glands have never been substantiated.[13]

III. PROGERIA (HUTCHINSON-GILFORD SYNDROME)

In 1866, Hutchinson described a 4-year-old boy with congenital alopecia, wrinkled "atrophic" skin, odd facies, joint contractures, and normal intelligence.[14] In 1904, Gilford reported a second case and suggested the name progeria for the syndrome.[15] In 1972, DeBusk reviewed the 60 cases of progeria then in the world literature, 36 males and 24 females, and tabulated their major manifestations.[16] Children appear completely normal at birth but soon develop profound growth failure, reduced subcutaneous fat especially on the face and limbs, striking facies, delayed and abnormal dentition, skeletal abnormalities such as dystrophic clavicles and coxa valga with joint contractures and a "horse-riding stance," and rapidly progressive atherosclerotic cardiovascular disease. After the first months of life, the clinical appearance is that of a "plucked bird" with a disproportionately large cranium and a relatively small face, prominent eyes and scalp veins, very sparse to absent scalp hair, frequently absent eyebrows and eyelashes, patent fontanels, centrofacial cyanosis, high-pitched voice, thin lips, and "beaked" nose (Plate 7).* Sexual maturation does not occur.

Like the rest of the body, the skin is usually unremarkable at birth, although generalized nonpitting edema suggestive of scleroderma has been reported.[17] Abnormalities evolve rapidly after several months of normal development, coincident with growth failure. By the second year, the skin is described as thin, dry, taut, and shiny in some areas, but lax and wrinkled in others. There is striking loss of subcutaneous fat, a prominent venous pattern, and easy bruising. Eccrine sweating is diminished. After several years, progressive irregular hyperpigmentation develops, most prominent in sun-exposed areas. Thickened sclerotic areas, usually on the lower trunk or thighs, have been reported in some patients; the nipples are occasionally hypoplastic. Generalized alopecia often begins in the first year, occasionally at birth, and is always marked by the end of the second year. The few remaining hairs are white or blond, very fine and "fuzzy," regardless of the original color and texture. Body hair, as well as scalp and facial hair, are affected. Fingernails and toenails have been described as short, thin, and dystrophic in the majority of reported cases. Koilonychia and onychogryposis have also been noted.

The prominence of skin changes in progeria is demonstrated by the fact that, despite marked growth retardation, 12 of 40 patients for whom such data are available were first brought to medical attention primarily because of alopecia or abnormal skin.[16] Certain histologic findings increase the resemblance of progeria to true premature aging. An autopsy report of two patients who died at ages 11 and 17 years with congestive heart failure revealed that both has extensive interstitial and focal myocardial fibrosis or necrosis with calcification of the mitral valve leaflets, and extensive lipofuscin ("age pigment") deposition in the brain, kidneys, adrenal glands, liver, testes, and heart,[18] all findings characteristic of elderly adults.

An early attempt to investigate the presumably deranged metabolism in progeria included studies of skin collagen from two unrelated patients aged 6 and 9 years.[22] Progeria collagen showed a higher shrinkage temperature at both low and high loads than did age-matched and normal adult collagen and a return to its original length after cooling, not attained in the controls. There was a smaller acid-soluble collagen fraction in the progeria specimens than in controls, but this result was also obtained in a pituitary dwarf, suggesting to the investigators that the finding reflected only very slow growth rather than a defect specific to progeria.

A histologic study of sclerodermatous skin from the abdomen of a boy with progeria revealed progressive hyalinization of dermal collagen and loss of subcutaneous fat over a 6-year period indistinguishable from scleroderma.[23] Scanning electron micrographs of residual hair shafts revealed unusual longitudinal depressions with minor cuticular defects.

Evidence for autosomal recessive inheritance of progeria is strong, with consanguinity reported in 3 of 19 known pedigrees and a high incidence of spontaneous abortion in affected

---

* Plate 7 appears after page 100.

families. An incidence of 1 per 8 million live births has been calculated.[16] Etiology is unknown. There is no support for early hypotheses of endocrine dysfunction or "hypermetabolism,"[19] and the suggestions that progeria is either due to vitamin E deficiency[20] or that its skin changes are improved by treatment with vitamin E[21] are without objective support.

IV. ACROGERIA

Acrogeria is a rare, presumably autosomal recessive disease, first described in two siblings by Grottron in the German literature.[24] In the ensuing 50 years, five additional cases have been reported.[24,25] Patients exhibit thin, dry, wrinkled skin with easy bruising and absence of subcutaneous fat, prominent venous pattern, and, in some cases, telangienctasia and mottled pigmentation (poikiloderma). The changes are most striking over the hands, feet, and distal 5 cm of the limbs, but subtly present over the trunk as well. Nails are dystrophic. The face is "pinched," and micrognathia is a feature in at least some patients. These cutaneous abnormalities may be detectable at birth and are usually prominent within the first year of life. The three patients described by Gilkes et al.[24] had low birthweight and persistent small stature. General health and life expectancy are said to be normal.

V. METAGERIA

The term metageria was coined by Gilkes et al.[24] to describe two unrelated patients with "premature aging," one male and one female, whose disease did not correspond to any previously described entity. From early childhood both were tall and thin with almost total absence of subcutaneous fat and distinctive thin "pinched" facies. At puberty, diffuse mottled hyperpigmentation developed, accompanied in one case by telangiectasia and Raynaud phenomenon. In this case, the combination of acral vasopasm and "very poor peripheral circulation" resulted in large chronic foot ulcers and gangrene bilaterally, requiring amputations at age 23 years. The skin was described as "atrophic" but soft, unlike that in scleroderma. Hair was very fine but normal in amount and color when examined at ages 20 to 25 years. The patients developed symptomatic diabetes mellitus at ages 17 and 20 years; no other endocrinopathy was apparent. At the time of the case report, one patient had died of unspecified causes at age 25 years.

Differences and similarities characterizing metageria, acrogeria, progeria, and Werner syndrome are summarized in Table 3.

VI. ROTHMUND SYNDROME

In 1868, Rothmund, an ophthalmologist, reported five patients from three inbred families of a remote German village who had childhood cataracts as well as atrophic, hyperpigmented, and telangiectatic skin.[6] In 1936, Thomson reported similar cases and proposed the name poikiloderma congenitale[26] for the syndrome which now frequently bears his name as well.

Abnormalities are usually noted in infancy. Affected individuals have short stature, cataracts, characteristic facies, skeletal abnormalities, small hands, hypogonadism, faulty dentition, sparse or absent eyebrows and eyelashes, dystrophic nails, poikiloderma, and photosensitivity sometimes associated with epidermal malignancies. Most patients also exhibit premature greying and loss of hair.[6,27]

The first skin lesions have been described as "red spots," detectable at approximately 3 months of age. Patients subsequently develop irregular hyperpigmentation, depigmented scars, scaling, striae, and livedo reticularis. The skin is thin but pliable, never sclerotic.[6] Available reports do not specify whether the poikilodermatous changes are accentuated in sun-exposed areas.

Table 3
CLINICAL FEATURES OF SELECTED AGING SYNDROMES WITH MAJOR CUTANEOUS MANIFESTATIONS

	Werner syndrome	Progeria	Acrogeria	Metageria
Onset of signs and symptoms	2nd decade	1st year of life	Birth	Birth
Diabetes mellitus	Mild, onset in 3rd-4th decade	Not a consistent feature	None	Onset in 2nd decade
Cardiovascular disease	Atherosclerosis with severe peripheral vascular disease, diffuse calcification, and myocardial infarction	Severe generalized atherosclerosis, interstitial and focal myocardial fibrosis, coronary artery disease with myocardial infarction	None	Early atherosclerosis, vascular calcification
Skeletal abnormalities	Osteoporosis, soft tissue calcification, short stature beginning in adolescence	Craniofacial disproportion, periarticular fibrosis, hypoplastic mandible, dystrophic short clavicles, short stature beginning at birth	Short stature	Tall stature
Secondary sexual characteristecs	Reduced fertility, scanty pubic hair, poor libido, early menopause.	Absence of sexual maturation	Normal	Normal
Life span	47 years average	13 years average	Normal	Probably reduced

Adapted from Gilkes, J. J. H., Sharvill, D. E., and Wells, R. S., *Br. J. Dermatol.*, 91, 243, 1974.

VII. COCKAYNE SYNDROME

In 1936, Cockayne reported a brother and sister with dwarfism, retinal atrophy, and deafness.[28] The 20 additional cases now reported outline a syndrome which includes "senile appearance" in childhood due to diffuse loss of subcutaneous fat; microcephaly, frequent progressive mental retardation, blindness, deafness, and other neurologic abnormalities; osteoporosis and other bony changes; photosensitivity; and occasional endocrine abnormalities.[1,27] Cockayne syndrome and xeroderma pigmentosum, both rare diseases, have been reported to co-exist in at least one patient.[29,30] Life expectancy is presumably much reduced, but few data are available.

VIII. GENERALIZED LIPODYSTROPHY

Generalized lipodystrophy, first described in 1928, has since been recognized as a distinct clinical entity, although its features may vary considerably among patients.[31] Hereditary lipodystrophy (Seip syndrome), an autosomal recessive disorder, is often classified among the premature aging syndromes[1,24] because the absence of subcutaneous fat gives an "aged" appearance to affected children, and because its features include diabetes mellitus, hypertension, and vascular disease. The cutaneous findings, however, are coarse dry skin, acanthosis nigricans, and hypertrichosis,[31] rather than "premature aging."

IX. TRISOMY 21 (DOWN SYNDROME)

Down syndrome is the most common chromosome aneuploidy and major congenital malformation of man.[27] The incidence is 1 per 660 live births; Down syndrome accounts for approximately one-third of patients institutionalized because of mental deficiency.

The resemblance to accelerated aging is not immediately obvious. Indeed, Down syndrome had been little studied from a gerontologic perspective until Martin's multifactorial analysis[1] revealed that this disorder regularly includes more features of "normal aging" than any of the classic aging syndromes, including Werner syndrome and progeria (15 vs. 12 and 10, respectively). The cited features are an increased incidence of autoimmune diseases and malignancy, premature greying or loss of hair, well-documented progressive dementia characterized histologically by the neurofibrillary tangles also found in routine "senile dementia," amyloid and lipofuscin deposition in many organs, diabetes mellitus, premature development of cataracts and cardiovascular disease, and a predominantly truncal distribution of fat.[1] Life span is shortened, even if neonatal deaths are excluded.[27]

Cutaneous features are laxity, xerosis, and according to some investigators, "atrophy," as well as the premature canities mentioned above.[27]

X. DIABETES MELLITUS

Diabetes mellitus, a common and complex disorder, is classified by some as a syndrome of premature aging because diabetics as a group experience geriatric disorders such as atherosclerosis and cataracts at a relatively early age and have a reduced life expectancy.[27] Diabetes mellitus has been cited as manifesting premature "skin atrophy" as "hair loss and/ or greying or both,"[27] although these features have never been noted in the dermatologic literature.

XI. MISCELLANEOUS

In addition to the more classic syndromes discussed above, there is a single case report of a patient with markedly accelerated wrinkling or "aging" of her skin on one half of the body only, first noted at age 60 years and most striking on the face and dorsum of the hand, chronically sun-exposed areas.[32] Histologic studies revealed a decrease in elastic tissue. The basic etiology could not be ascertained, and the disorder appeared to be restricted to the skin.

XII. LABORATORY STUDIES

To date, virtually all laboratory investigations of the premature aging syndromes have used cultured fibroblasts, in most instances derived from the skin.[33]

A. Studies of Cellular Growth Potential

Soon after Hayflick established that human diploid fibroblasts have a finite reproducible culture life span which is inversely proportional to the donor's age[34] and proposed in vitro aging of cultured fibroblasts as a model for in vivo aging of the entire organism, Martin et al. reported that the life span of fibroblasts cultured from the skin of four patients with Werner syndrome fell more than two standard deviations below the mean for age-matched control fibroblasts.[35,36] Single patients with progeria and Rothmund syndrome, studied in the same laboratory, each ranked 23 to 26 in fibroblast growth potential for the respective age cohorts when compared to clinically normal subjects.[36] Goldstein has reported an even more markedly reduced fibroblast growth potential in progeria, achieving only two subcultures vs. 20 to 30 for controls.[37] Studies of fibroblasts from three additional progeria patients revealed decreased mitotic activity, rate of outgrowth from explants, DNA synthesis, and cloning efficiency compared to those of controls, all consistent with accelerated aging in vitro, although culture life span was not determined.[38] More recently, progeria fibroblasts have been shown to be poorly responsive to an insulin-like activity which stimulates growth in culture, requiring two to three times as much mitogen to achieve the same DNA synthesis as age-matched control fibroblasts.[39] Dermal fibroblasts from patients with Cockayne syndrome have a marked decrease in colony forming efficiency after UV irradiation compared to controls, although thymine dimer repair appears normal.[40]

All of the premature aging syndromes studied to date have manifested a similar reduction in fibroblast growth potential in vitro. These include Down syndrome,[41,42] diabetes mellitus,[43] and other syndromes not included in this discussion.[27] Overall, the severity of fibroblast growth failure correlates with the severity of clinical "aging," supporting the hypothesis that in vitro cellular growth potential in some way reflects the donor's physiologic age.

B. Studies of Cellular Proteins

Glucose-6-phosphate dehydrogenase (G6PD) and 6-phosphogluconic acid dehydrogenase (6PGD), enzymes of the hexose monophosphate shunt, can be assayed in cultured fibroblasts and have an increased heat-labile fraction in late passage as compared to that in early passage cells,[44] a finding that is interpreted as a manifestation of in vitro aging. Hypoxanthineguanine phosphoribosyltransferase (HGPRT), an enzyme involved in purine metabolism, and G6PD are known to alter during the normal 4-month "aging" process of circulating human erythrocytes.[45,46]

Studies of these three enzymes (G6PD, 6-PGD, and HGPRT) in cultured skin fibroblasts of patients with both progeria[47] and Werner syndrome[48-50] have revealed markedly increased heat-labile fractions throughout the culture life span, with a proportionate decrease in each enzyme's specific activity.[51] These data have been used to suggest a close relationship between normal aging and the pathophysiology of these recessive diseases, as well as a possible disease mechanism.

Cultured fibroblasts from patients with progeria and Rothmund syndrome have been reported to show markedly increased affinity of surface insulin receptors for native insulin when compared to age-matched controls.[52] This may be seen as an analogy to normal aging with its nearly fourfold increase in insulin binding between the first and seventh decades,[52] and corresponds to the clinical findings of relative insulin resistance in both progeria[22] and normal aging.[52a] More recently, cultured dermal fibroblasts from a progeric patient were shown to require two to threefold higher concentrations of plasma-derived insulin-like activity (ILA) in order to stimulate 50 and 95% of their maximal thymidine uptake (DNA synthesis), compared to fibroblasts from age-matched normal children or from young adults.[52a] Old adult fibroblasts required intermediate concentrations to achieve equivalent stimulation of DNA synthesis. Similarly, stimulation of glucose uptake in response to a fixed ILA concentration was less for progeric fibroblasts than for either age-matched or adult controls at early passage. This decreased responsiveness was due to higher basal rates of glucose uptake for progeric cells; absolute values for ILA-stimulated uptake were comparable. In both assays, progeric fibroblasts resembled early passage fibroblasts from old donors and late passage fibroblasts from all donor groups, i.e., cells "aged" in vivo or in vitro.

Other molecular abnormalities in cells cultured from patients with progeria and Werner syndrome, for which no corresponding normally age-associated change is yet recognized, include a marked-to-moderate decrease in the number of surface-membrane HLA antigens[27] and much increased activity of a tissue-derived procoagulant which has been postulated to predispose these patients to accelerated atherosclerosis.[53] Decreased mobility of cell membrane receptors has been reported in patients with Down syndrome and in normal elderly subjects.[54]

Decreased repair of single-strand DNA breaks following ionizing radiation was reported by one group for certain progeria fibroblast strains,[55,56] but could not be confirmed by three other groups.[27] A similar defect of DNA repair has been reported for Cockayne and Rothmund syndrome fibroblasts.[57,58] Postirradiation DNA repair appears completely normal in Werner syndrome,[27] although cultured fibroblasts may have reduced karyotype stability[59] and decreased rate of DNA replication.[60] Such reductions in DNA repair capacity or stability might increase the rate of genomic deterioration and, in turn, the rate of cellular aging.

XIII. CONCLUSIONS

Although all the premature aging syndromes manifest certain features suggestive of accelerated aging, none closely mimics the normal aging process. The distribution, specific character, and developmental sequence of pathologic findings diverge from those of normal aging for most organ systems in each syndrome. Furthermore, in each disorder many of the accepted features of normal aging are lacking. These discrepancies are at least as pronounced in the skin as in the other involved organ systems.

Most of the premature aging syndromes are transmitted by autosomal recessive genes, yet have multiple features that are difficult or impossible to attribute to a single defective enzyme or other protein structure. This suggests that the syndromes may be due to errors in the regulation of various metabolic pathways and argues in favor of an explicit genetic program for aging. The frequency and variety of cutaneous abnormalities in these complex syndromes emphasize the integral relationship of the skin to the rest of the body and the potential value of the skin as a tissue source for studies of underlying disease mechanisms.

The relatively recent application of tissue culture technology to the study of progeria, Werner syndrome, and other premature aging syndromes has already yielded considerable data, offering the hope that our understanding of these diseases may increase rapidly in the coming decades.

REFERENCES

1. **Martin, G. M.,** Genetic syndromes in man with potential relevance to the pathobiology of aging, in *Genetic Effects of Aging,* Bergsma, D. and Harrison, D. E., Eds., Alan R. Liss, the National Foundation-March of Dimes, New York, 1978.
2. **Selmanowitz, V. J., Rizer, R. L., and Orentreich, N.,** Aging of the skin and its appendages, in *Handbook of the Biology of Aging,* Finch, C. E. and Hayflick, L., Eds., Van Nostrand Reinhold, New York, 1977, 496.
3. **Gilchrest, B. A.,** Aging of the skin, in *Pathophysiology of the Skin,* Baden, H. P. and Soter, N. A., Eds., McGraw-Hill, New York, 1983, in press.
4. **Gilchrest, B. A.,** Age-associated changes in the skin: overview and clinical relevance, *J. Am. Gerontol. Soc.,* 30, 139, 1982.
5. **Werner, O.,** *Uber Katarakt in Verbindung mit Schlerodermie,* Schmidt et Klaunig, Kiel, Germany, 1904.
6. **Thannahauser, S. J.,** Werner's syndrome (progeria of the adult) and Rothmund's syndrome: two types of closely related heredofamilial atrophic dermatoses with juvenile cataracts and endocrine features: a critical study with five new cases, *Ann. Intern. Med.,* 23, 559, 1945.
7. **Epstein, C. J., Martin, G. M., Schultz, A. L., and Motulsky, A. G.,** Werner's syndrome: a review of its symptomatology, natural history, pathologic features, genetics, and relationship to the natural aging process, *Medicine,* 45, 177, 1966.
8. **Fleischmajer, R. and Nedwich, A.,** Werner's syndrome, *Am. J. Med.,* 54, 111, 1973.
9. **Zalla, J. A.,** Werner's syndrome, *Cutis,* 25, 275, 1980.

10. **Bjornberg, A.,** Werner's syndrome and malignancy, *Acta Derm. Venereol. (Stockh),* 56, 149, 1976.
11. **Rabbiosi, G. and Borroni, G.,** Werner's syndrome: seven cases in one family, *Dermatologica,* 158, 355, 1979.
12. **Hrabko, R. P., Milgrom, H., and Schwartz, R. A.,** Werner's syndrome with associated malignant neoplasm, *Arch. Dermatol.,* 118, 106, 1982.
13. **Alberti, K. G., Young, J. D., and Hockaday, T. D.,** Werner's syndrome: metabolic observations, *Proc. Roy. Soc. Med.,* 67, 36, 1974.
14. **Hutchinson, J.,** Congenital absence of hair and mammary glands with atrophic condition of the skin and its appendages, *Med. Chir. Trans.,* 69, 473, 1886.
15. **Gilford, H.,** Progeria: a form of senilism, *Practitioner,* 73, 188, 1904.
16. **DeBusk, F. L.,** The Hutchinson-Gilford progeria syndrome, *J. Pediatr.,* 80, 697, 1972.
17. **Runge, P., Asnis, M. S., Brumley, G. W., and Grossman, H.,** Hutchinson-Gilford progeria syndrome, *South. Med. J.,* 71, 877, 1978.
18. **Reichel, W. and Garcia-Brunel, R.,** Pathologic findings in progeria: myocardial fibrosis and lipofuscin pigment, *Am. J. Clin. Pathol.,* 53, 243, 1970.
19. **Atkins, L.,** Progeria. Report of a case with post-mortem findings, *N. Engl. J. Med.,* 250, 1065, 1954.
20. **Ayres, S., Jr. and Mihan, R.,** Letter: progeria: a possible therapeutic approach, *JAMA,* 227, 1381, 1974.
21. **Ayres, S., Jr. and Mihan, R.,** Vitamin E and dermatology, *Cutis,* 16, 1017, 1975.
22. **Villee, D. B., Nichols, G., Jr., and Talbot, N. B.,** Metabolic studies in two boys with classical progeria, *Pediatrics,* 43, 207, 1969.
23. **Fleischmajer, R., and Nedwich, A.,** Progeria (Hutchinson-Gilford), *Arch. Dermatol.,* 107, 253, 1973.
24. **Gilkes, J. J. H., Sharvill, D. E., and Wells, R. S.,** The premature aging syndromes. Report of eight cases and description of a new entity named metageria, *Br. J. Dermatol.,* 91, 243, 1974.
25. **Calvert, H. T.,** Acrogeria (Gottron type), *Br. J. Dermatol.,* 69, 69, 1957.
26. **Thomson, M. S.,** Poikiloderma congenitale, *Br. J. Dermatol.,* 48, 221, 1936.
27. **Goldstein, S.,** Human genetic disorders that feature premature onset and accelerated progression of biological aging, in *The Genetics of Aging,* Schneider, E. L., Ed., Plenum Press, New York, 1978, 171.
28. **Cockayne, E. A.,** Dwarfism with retinal atrophy and deafness, *Arch. Dis. Child.,* 11, 1, 1936.
29. **Robbins, J. H., Kraemer, K. H., Lutzner, M. A., Festoff, B. W., and Coon, H. G.,** Xeroderma pigmatosum: an inherited disease with sun sensitivity, multiple cutaneous neoplasms, and abnormal DNA repair, *Ann. Intern. Med.,* 80, 221, 1974.
30. **Dupuy, J. M. and Lafforet, D.,** Xeroderma pigmentosum and Cockayne syndrome (letter), *Pediatrics,* 61, 675, 1978.
31. **Senior, B. and Gellis, S. S.,** The syndromes of total lipodystrophy and of partial lipodystrophy, *Pediatrics,* 33, 593, 1964.
32. **Shelley, W. B. and Wood, M. G.,** Unilateral wrinkles — manifestation of unilateral elastic tissue defect, *Arch. Dermatol.,* 110, 775, 1974.
33. **Goldstein, S.,** Studies on age-related diseases in cultured skin fibroblasts, *J. Invest. Dermatol.,* 73, 19, 1979.
34. **Hayflick, L.,** The limited in vitro lifetime of human diploid cell strains, *Exp. Cell. Res.,* 37, 614, 1965.
35. **Martin, G. M., Gartler, S. M., Epstein, C. J., and Motulsky, A. G.,** Diminished lifespan of cultured cells in Werner's syndrome, *Fed Proc. Fed. Am. Soc. Exp. Biol.,* 24, 678, 1965.
36. **Martin, G. M., Sprague, C. A., and Epstein, C. J.,** Replicative life-span of cultivated human cells, *Lab. Invest.,* 23, 86, 1970.
37. **Goldstein, S.,** Life-span of cultured cells in progeria, *Lancet,* 1, 424, 1969.
38. **Danes, B. S.,** Progeria: a cell culture study on aging, *J. Clin. Invest.,* 50, 2000, 1971.
39. **Harley, C. B., Goldstein, S., Posner, B. I., and Guyda, H.,** Decreased sensitivity of old and progeric human fibroblasts to a preparation of factors with insulinlike activity, *J. Clin. Invest.,* 68, 988, 1981.
40. **Schmickel, R. D., Chu, E. H. Y., Trosko, J. E., and Chang, C. C.,** Cockayne syndrome: a cellular sensitivity to ultraviolet light, *Pediatrics,* 60, 135, 1977.
41. **Schneider, E. L. and Epstein, C. J.,** Replication rate and lifespan of cultured fibroblasts in Down's syndrome, *Proc. Soc. Exp. Biol. Med.,* 141, 1092, 1972.
42. **Boue, A., Boue, J., Cure, S., et al.,** In vitro cultivation of cells from aneuploid human embryos: initiation of cell lines and longevity of the cultures, *In Vitro,* 11, 409, 1975.
43. **Goldstein, S., Moerman, E. J., Soeldner, J. S., et al.,** Chronologic and physiologic age affect replicative life-span of fibroblasts from diabetic, prediabetic, and normal donors, *Science,* 199, 781, 1978.
44. **Holliday, R. and Tarrant, G. M.,** Altered enzymes in aging human fibroblasts, *Nature (London),* 238, 26, 1972.
45. **Fornaini, G., Leoncini, G., Segni, P., et al,** Relationship between age and properties of human and rabbit erythrocyte glucose-6-phosphate dehydrogenase, *Eur. J. Biochem.,* 7, 214, 1969.

46. **Yip, L. C., Dancis, J., Mathieson, B., et al.,** Age-induced changes in adenosine monophosphate: pyrophosphate phosphoribosyltransferase and inosine monophosphate: pyrophosphate phosphoribosyltransferase from normal and Lesch-Nyhan erythrocytes, *Biochemistry,* 13, 2558. 1974.

47. **Goldstein, S. and Moerman, E. J.,** Heat-labile enzymes in skin fibroblasts from subjects with progeria, *N. Engl. J. Med.,* 292, 1305, 1975.

48. **Goldstein, S. and Moerman, E. J.,** Heat-labile enzymes in Werner's syndrome fibroblasts, *Nature (London),* 255, 159, 1975.

49. **Goldstein, S. and Singal, D. P.,** Alteration of fibroblast gene products in vitro from a subject with Werner's syndrome, *Nature (London),* 251, 719, 1974.

50. **Holliday, R., Porterfield, J. S., and Gibbs, D. D.,** Premature aging and occurrence of altered enzyme in Werner's syndrome fibroblasts, *Nature (London),* 248, 762, 1974.

51. **Goldstein, S. and Moerman, E. J.,** Defective proteins in normal and abnormal human fibroblasts during aging in vitro, *Interdiscip. Top. Gerontol.,* 10, 24, 1976.

52. **Rosenbloom, A. L., Goldstein, S., and Yip, C. C.,** Insulin binding to cultured human fibroblasts increases with normal and precocious aging, *Science.* 193, 412, 1976.

52a. **DeFronzo, R. A.,** Glucose intolerance and aging. Evidence for tissue insensitivity to insulin, *Diabetes,* 28, 1095, 1979.

52b. **Harley, C. B., Goldstein, S., Posner, B. I., and Guyda, H.,** Decreased sensitivity of old and progeric human fibroblasts to a preparation of factors with insulinlike activity, *J. Clin. Invest.,* 68, 988, 1981.

53. **Goldstein, S. and Niewiarowski, S.,** Increased precoagulant activity in cultured fibroblasts from progeria and Werner's syndromes of premature aging, *Nature (London),* 260, 711, 1976.

54. **Naeim, F. and Walford, R. L.,** Disturbance of redistribution of surface membrane receptors on peripheral mononuclear cells of patients with Down's syndrome and of aged individuals, *J. Gerontol.,* 35, 650, 1980.

55. **Epstein, J., Williams, J. R., and Little, J. B.,** Deficient DNA repair in human progeroid cells, *Proc. Natl. Acad. Sci. U.S.A.,* 70, 977, 1973.

56. **Epstein, J., Williams, J. R., and Little, J. B.,** Rate of DNA repair in progeric and normal human fibroblasts, *Biochem. Biophys. Res. Commun.,* 59, 850, 1974.

57. **Schmickel, R. D., Chu, E. H. Y., and Troska, J.,** The definition of a cellular defect in two patients with Cockayne syndrome, *Pediatr. Res.,* 9, 317, 1975.

58. **Cleaver, J. E.,** DNA damage and repair in light-sensitive human skin disease, *J. Invest. Dermatol.,* 54, 181, 1970.

59. **Norwood, T. H., Hoehm, H., Salk, D., and Martin, G. M.,** Cellular aging in Werner's syndrome: a unique phenotype? *J. Invest. Dermatol.,* 73, 92, 1979.

60. **Nakao, Y., Kishihara, M., Yoshimi, H., Inoue, Y., Tanaka, K., Sakamoto, N., Matsukura, S., Imura, H., Ichihashi, M., and Fujiwara, Y.,** Werner's syndrome: in vivo and in vitro characteristics as a model of aging, *Am. J. Med.,* 65, 919, 1978.

61. **Riccardi, V., Hall, J., and Bauer, E.,** personal communication.

Chapter 6

AGING AND SKIN CANCER

I. INTRODUCTION

The clinical and investigative aspects of carcinogenesis constitute a vast literature, well beyond the capacity of a single chapter to review. This discussion will focus exclusively on the epidemiologic and possibly causal relationships between aging and cancer, with special emphasis on skin cancer.

II. EPIDEMIOLOGY

It is widely recognized that the incidence of malignant neoplasia increases with age in both animals and man.[1] A few malignancies, most notably prostatic carcinoma, occur very commonly in the elderly. In one large autopsy series, point prevalence in man for clinically detectable prostatic carcinoma increased from near zero at age 40 to approximately one-third at age 90 years, and the prevalence for microscopic foci of carcinoma in the gland from approximately 2% to an apparent plateau of nearly 50% by age 70 years.[2] The prevalence for clinically detectable cancer of all types (excluding basal cell carcinoma) showed a similar steep increase after age 40 years to approximately 40% at age 90 years in the same series.[2] If microscopic prostatic carcinoma and cutaneous basal cell carcinoma were included, the maximum prevalence approached 60 to 70%.

Two points regarding the increasing risk of malignancy with age deserve emphasis. First, although most individual ''adult'' malignancies (in contrast to ''childhood'' leukemias, neuroblastoma, etc.) demonstrate an increasing incidence (diagnosis rate) with age,[3,4] the absolute incidence of each malignancy with very few exceptions is low, usually well below 1% at any age.[5] Second, the relationship between most cancer incidence and adult age in the population is not linear but exponential, with very little increase in cancer rate during the third to fifth decades, and a very steep increase during the next 3 decades.[4,5] The most reliable data suggest that the point prevalence for human malignancies approximately doubles every 9 years until age 80, then increases only slightly thereafter.

The same pattern is apparent for skin cancer (Figure 1). The increasing incidence through-out adulthood for all three major cutaneous malignancies[6] — basal cell carcinoma, squamous cell carcinoma, and melanoma — require emphasis, as absolute incidence figures, uncor-rected for the size of each age cohort in the population, peak during the middle age and decline in the elderly.

Closer examination of the relationship between patient age and cancer incidence for the special case of nonmelanoma skin cancer yields a perhaps surprising phenomenon. Regardless of the absolute incidence figures, which vary more than threefold for the susceptible white population among geographic areas in the U.S.[7,8] depending on regional insolation (total annual solar UV irradiation at ground level),[7,8] the rate of increase in cancer incidence in each area is a function only of patient age, not of exposure to the presumed environmental carcinogen (Figure 2). Moreover, skin cancer first appears during the fourth decade in the white population (0.01% > age-specific incidence > 0.001%) in all geographic areas, again independent of sun exposure (Figure 3). These data appear to contradict experimental work demonstrating that exposure to higher doses of UV light or other known carcinogens is associated with an earlier onset as well as greater final yield for tumors in rodents.[9,9a] The different pattern apparent from the human epidemiologic data may reflect a different age-related vulnerability to photocarcinogenesis or simply the vagaries inherent in indirect meas-urement (regional UV fluence rather than the patients' actual UV exposures).

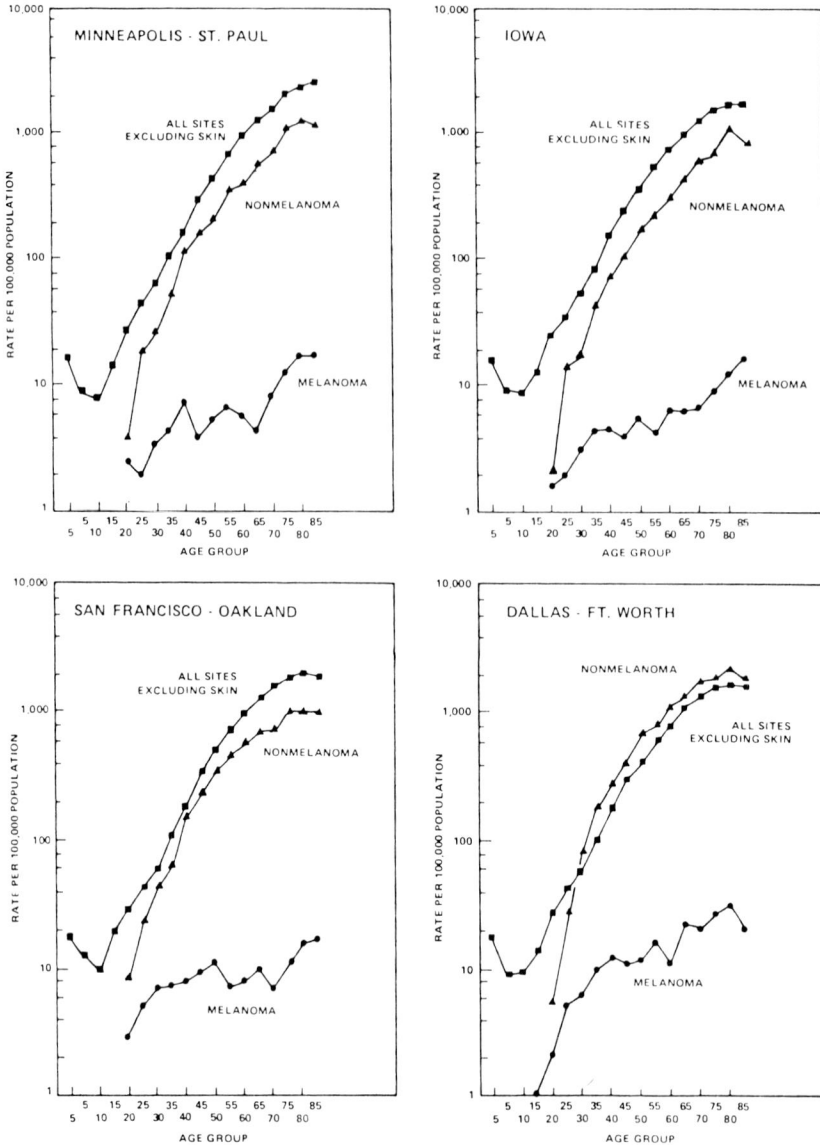

FIGURE 1. Age-specific cancer incidence among whites in four areas of the U.S. Note the striking similarity (a) between curves for all malignancies (excluding skin cancer) and nonmelanoma skin cancer, and (b) among families of curves in the different geographic areas. (From Scotto, J. and Fears, T. R., *Natl. Cancer Inst. Monogr.*, 50, 169, 1978. With permission.)

Finally, it is of interest to note that nonmelanoma skin cancer, which is undeniably related to sun exposure, i.e., can be attributed in most instances to a carcinogen, conforms almost exactly to the pattern of other presumably "spontaneous" malignancies (Figures 1 and 2). While this may be purely coincidental, it suggests that age-related systemic changes in part determine the expression of malignancy, regardless of other contributory factors.[9b]

III. AGE-RELATED RISK FACTORS FOR CANCER

Whether older individuals are at increased risk for carcinogenesis following an "inciting

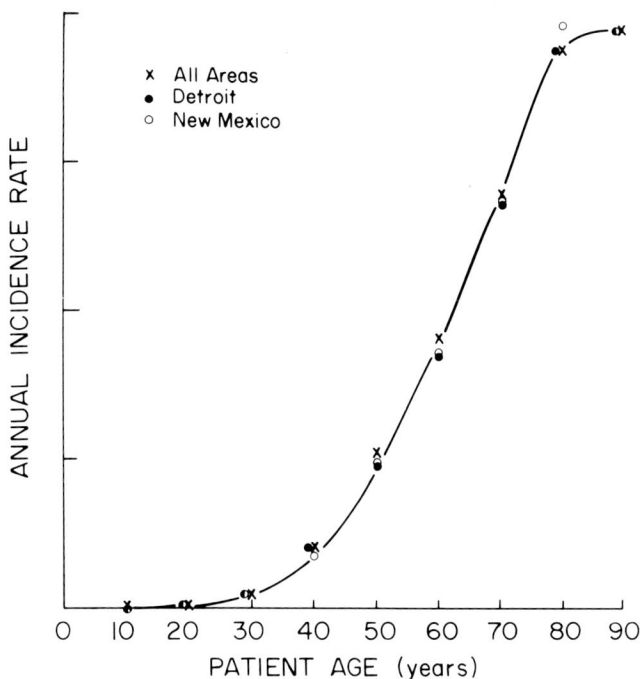

FIGURE 2. Relationship between patient age and cancer incidence. The sigmoid plot of incidence vs. age is typical of that observed in several autopsy studies of human malignancy.[2-5] The graphed symbols represent the age-specific incidence for nonmelanoma skin cancer reported in 1977 to 1978 for the white U.S. population in eight geographic areas:[8] (x) average for all 8 areas, (○) New Mexico, an area of high insolation and high skin cancer rate, and (●) Detroit, an area of low insolation and low skin cancer rate. Incidence figures are normalized to a single maximal value for the oldest available group (85 +) in each area and the remaining incidences for the 35 to 44, 45 to 54, 55 to 64, 65 to 74, and 75 to 84 year-old groups are reported as a percent of this maximal value. Absolute age-adjusted crude rates per 100,000 population are 232.6 overall, 336.7 in New Mexico, and 135.6 in Detroit.[8] Despite a more than threefold range of cancer incidence among the areas surveyed, attributed to their varying insolation, the relationships between incidence and patient age are remarkably similar. These virtually identical curves suggest that the major effect of UV irradiation is to increase an inherent age-related predisposition to develop skin cancer.

event'' such as exposure to a carcinogen, remains unclear. Unequivocal experiments are difficult to design, as most carcinogens require relatively long induction times and animals initiated in old age therefore die before developing cancers.

In one innovative study,[10] Ebbesen grafted skin from mice age 2 months and 14 months to syngeneic young mice, then applied dimethylbenz(a)anthracene (DMBA) to the grafted skin. Carcinomas (diagnosed histologically and by their ability to grow intraperitoneally in new hosts) developed in 16/41 (39%) of the old grafts and in 5/41 (12%) of the young grafts ($p < 0.001$) within 8 months. There was no difference in the graft size between the two groups. However, DMBA-treated mice bearing old skin grafts also had a slightly higher incidence of noncutaneous tumors (leukemias and reticulosarcomas) than did those bearing young skin grafts, raising the possibility of greater DMBA penetration through old skin with consequently greater carcinogen exposure in this group. Other investigators have found the incidence of skin tumors in mice following repeated application of benzo(a)pyrene varies

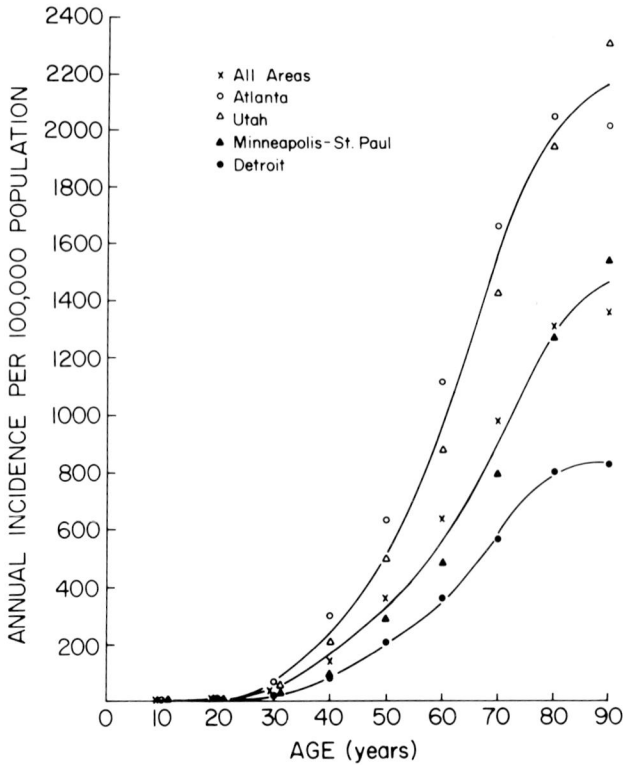

FIGURE 3.   Annual age-specific incidence rates for nonmelanoma skin cancer for whites in various geographic areas. Data are graphed for representative areas of low incidence (Detroit), intermediate incidence (Minneapolis-St. Paul), and high incidence (Atlanta and Utah), and for the average of all eight surveyed areas.[8] Curves are derived from the same data as in Figure 2, graphed as absolute values rather than as normalized values.

only with duration of exposure to the carcinogens, not with age of the animal, within the limits imposed by this experimental design.[11]

Forbes, Davies, and Urbach reported a delayed onset and decreased peak incidence for murine skin tumors induced by daily UVB irradiation when the same total dose was given as 25% from the 6th to 11th week of life and 75% from the 11th to 16th week than if the dose were given in the reverse manner.[12] Similarly, mice irradiated for 10 weeks beginning at age 6 weeks developed slightly more tumors than mice irradiated in the same way beginning at age 16 weeks. From these data, the authors conclude that older animals are less susceptible to photocarcinogenesis. Unfortunately, the younger mice were immature, while the older mice were mature at the onset of irradiation, so that the effect of adult aging was not examined. Furthermore, as noted by the authors, age-associated changes other than cellular susceptibility to transformation, such as protective stratum corneum thickness, might have contributed to their results.[12]

IV. AGING, CARCINOGENESIS, AND DNA REPAIR

Cellular DNA, the repository of all cellular programs, is widely assumed to participate in the aging process in some capacity,[13-16] and is certainly involved in the malignant transformation of cells. Furthermore, the rate and extent of repair for at least UV-induced DNA damage is closely correlated with maximum attainable life span in seven mammalian species ranging from shrews and mice to man,[17] strengthening the suspicion that DNA repair capacity is a determinant in the rate of aging. Whether aging and oncogenesis are linked in any more direct manner remains a matter of conjecture, however.

DNA repair is perhaps especially important in the skin, where cells are subject not only to endogenous baseline damage to their genetic material, but to continuous bombardment from the environment. The clinical implications for aging skin are twofold. First, the aging process in skin may affect its DNA repair capacity, so that a given insult may produce more (or less) damage in older individuals. Second, environmental influences on the skin may actually accelerate (or retard) the aging process.

Investigators have noted that exposure to ionizing radiation or mutagens known to damage DNA and increase carcinogenesis may shorten an organism's life span, even in the absence of malignancies,[18-20] but the changes produced differ quantitatively and qualitatively from normal aging, and of the genetic syndromes associated with abnormal DNA repair and malignancy, few entail ''premature aging'' and none closely mimics accelerated normal aging.[21] Recent studies have attempted to address the possible causal relationship between aging and DNA fidelity/oncogenesis in tissue culture systems utilizing a variety of fibroblast strains. In vitro aging (early vs. late passage cells) has been investigated more extensively than in vivo aging (early passage cells from young vs. old tissue donors).

Early passage and late passage (senescent) WI-38 cells have been shown equally capable of supporting the replication of three different viruses.[22] The virus' rate of production and yield per cell were comparable at early and late passage, and further data argue strongly against age-associated decline in the fidelity of DNA replication or translation: early and late passage cells produced virus with nearly identical specific infectivity, thermal inactivation kinetics (suggesting an absence of faulty structural proteins), and mutation rates.[22]

UV-induced unscheduled DNA synthesis, indicative of repair, has been found to decline in human skin fibroblasts[23] and fetal lung fibroblasts[24-26] at the very end of their in vitro life span. Hart and Setlow, in further examining the possible relation between in vitro senescence and loss of DNA repair capacity, found that the percentage of cultured WI-38 cells undergoing scheduled DNA synthesis progressively declines from essentially 100% at early passage to less than 10% at the end of their in vitro life span[25] (confirming the results of earlier investigators[27]) and that, in general, only those cells remaining in the dividing pool (i.e., capable of scheduled DNA synthesis) performed normal amounts of unscheduled DNA synthesis following UV irradiation.[25] The ability to rejoin single-strand breaks also appears to decrease during in vitro senescence for cultured human dermal fibroblasts,[28-30] human fetal lung fibroblasts,[31] mouse embryo fibroblasts,[32] and chick fibroblasts,[33] although this has not been consistently observed for WI-38 cells.[34-35] Overall, the data suggest that compromised DNA repair is not a striking feature of cellular senescence in vitro and is more likely to result from metabolic and proliferative derangements in late passage cells than to cause them.[17,36] The data do not, however, preclude an increasing risk of mutation or carcinogenesis during in vitro aging.

The few studies that have examined DNA repair capacity for dermal fibroblasts as a function of donor age have yielded apparently conflicting results. Goldstein found no difference in short-term cell survival following UV irradiation of early passage fibroblasts of fetal, newborn, young adult and old adult origin;[23] while Sbano et al. have reported an age-related decline in DNA excision repair for fibroblasts obtained from both habitually exposed and nonexposed areas in a small group of adult subjects aged 50 to 80 years.[37] The latter study, designed to investigate factors predisposing to photocarcinogenesis, also found consistently higher levels of repair in cultures derived from sun-exposed skin and less repair in cultures derived from subjects with actinic keratoses than in those from approximately age-matched controls without precancerous skin lesions. These interesting results require confirmation in groups sufficiently large to permit statistical validation.

The postulated reduction in DNA repair capacity among patients with actinic keratoses, if substantiated, may not be restricted to cells in the skin. Lymphocytes from 10 such patients, aged 53 to 81 years, were reported to have a statistically lower level of UV-induced DNA repair synthesis than approximately age-matched control subjects,[38] although no correlation between DNA repair and donor age was apparent in either group.[38] A similar study of UV-induced DNA repair capacity in lymphocytes from 18 patients with actinic keratoses and 18 age-matched controls measured an approximately 50% reduction in the former group.[39] The presentation of data did not permit examination of possible age-related changes in DNA repair for either group, however. Both groups of authors conclude that patients with actinic keratoses may be genetically predisposed to suffer sun damage to their skin, in a manner analogous to patients with xeroderma pigmentosum.

Schneider and co-workers have reported that human dermal fibroblasts derived from 65 to 80-year-old vs. 20 to 33-year-old adult donors have similar rates of spontaneous sister chromatid exchange (SCE) throughout their in vitro life span, but that early passage cells from old donors manifest up to 25 to 30% fewer SCE than do early cells from young donors exposed to the mutagens mitomycin C or *N*-acetoxy-2-acetylaminofluorene (AAAF).[40] The same laboratory has also demonstrated a reduction in mutagen-induced SCE for human fetal lung fibroblasts (WI-38 and IMR-90) at late vs. early passage and for old vs. young rodent bone marrow cells examined in vivo.[42] The authors note that should SCE indeed indicate DNA repair, these data strongly suggest that DNA repair in response to chemical mutagen exposure declines during aging both in vitro and in vivo.

Recent advances in keratinocyte culture techniques have permitted investigation of DNA repair capacity in this second cell type. Initial studies suggest that DNA repair of cultured keratinocytes following UV (254 nm) irradiation is comparable in efficiency and time course to that of dermal fibroblasts.[43,44] In the first study examining the effect of keratinocyte donor age on DNA repair capacity, Liu, Parsons, and Hanawalt employed a 5-bromodeoxyuridine density-labeling method to assess UV-induced excision repair.[45] Cultured epidermal keratinocytes obtained at autopsy from infants and adults (mean age 60 years, maximum age 90 years) demonstrated identical degrees of inhibition of semiconservative DNA replication over 24 hr in response to increasing UV doses, with more than 90% inhibition following a 50 J/cm^2 dose which detached approximately half the keratinocytes from the culture dishes at 24 hr. Evidence of "unscheduled" repair replication was reported to be maximal at this dose. A comparison of repair replication between one infant and two adult cultures performed after a 13 J/cm^2 dose during the second culture week revealed identical time courses over 24 hr when examined as percent of the final value, with 70% of total repair occurring within 6 hr after irradiation. No decline in repair capacity was noted for an adult strain studied both at 11 days while still proliferating in culture and at 25 days during the "decay phase" when the cultures were dying in this system. The authors conclude that, as in the case of cultured human fibroblasts, there is little evidence for decreased DNA repair capacity during in vivo or in vitro aging of cultured epidermal keratinocytes. They do note that DNA repair for human skin in vivo appears to be considerably faster than that observed in their cultures,[46] suggesting (as in some other situations) that in vitro systems may not accurately reflect in vivo cellular capacities.

The possible causal relationships between failure of DNA repair mechanisms and oncogenesis or aging have also been suggested based on studies of patients with xeroderma pigmentosum (XP), an autosomal recessive disorder characterized by a more than 1000-fold increase in incidence of cutaneous malignancies and a profound deficiency of DNA repair following UV-irradiation.[47] XP patients are said to manifest "premature aging" of the skin, although published descriptions are lacking, and the observed changes more probably reflect accelerated sun-damage or "dermatoheliosis," a clinical syndrome synonymous in the public mind with cutaneous aging. However, some patients are also said to have pathologic changes in the central nervous system which resemble those asociated with normal aging. Most XP patients in the past died young as a consequence of metastatic malignancy. Early diagnosis and virtually complete sun avoidance are now permitting a small number of patients to reach adulthood with little cutaneous change. Life span data for these individuals lacking normal DNA repair capacity but spared fatal UV-induced cancers will be of great theoretic interest.

V. OTHER POSSIBLE AGE-ASSOCIATED RISK FACTORS

Table 1 lists factors which have been postulated to contribute to the development of skin cancer in the elderly.

Cumulative exposure to carcinogens and increased induction time following exposure are relevant considerations for virtually all human cancers, although the role of environmental carcinogens is better understood for the skin than for most organ systems. Evidence for decreased DNA repair capacity with aging is discussed above.

A decrease in cell-mediated immunity with advancing age is well documented in both animals and man.[48] Burnet,[49] who originated the concept of immunologic surveillance, and many others[48,50] have suggested that loss of cell-mediated immunity renders the elderly less capable of detecting and destroying transformed cells as they arise and hence permits the clinical expression of malignancy. Decreased cutaneous expression of cell-mediated immunity has been observed in several studies: comparison between two groups of 45 healthy volunteers indicated that 70% of those younger than 80 years reacted to at least one of five standard recall antigens, whereas only 24% of the octagenarians did.[51] Similarly, in a study of 116 normal subjects, 94% of those less than 70 years could be sensitized to dinitro-chlorobenzene (DNCB) vs. 69% of those 70 years or older.[52] Moreover, in a separate study, the response to intradermal DNCB injection in nine previously sensitized subjects was significantly less ($p < 0.05$) in clinically sun-damaged, elastotic skin of the posterior neck than in adjacent sun-protected back skin.[53] No difference in DNCB responses between neck and back skin was observed in six control subjects lacking clinical stigmata of sun damage. Intradermal injection of candidin, mumps, and PPD antigens yields larger areas of induration in the sun-protected sites than in the sun-damaged sites ($p < 0.05$) in the same subjects. Reaction to application of the irritant benzalkonium chloride was identical in both sites, implying equal capacity for manifesting inflammation. The authors conclude that the decreased delayed hypersensitivity observed in sun-damaged sites was due to a local immunologic defect. Although the precise nature of this defect is unknown, UV irradiation has been shown to profoundly alter and/or deplete epidermal Langerhans cells (LC), the cell presumably responsible for antigen recognition in the skin, in both experimental animals and man. Toews, Bergstresser, and Streilein first demonstrated that repeated UV irradiation of mouse skin greatly reduced the number of LC as recognized by ATPase surface markers and that the irradiated LC-depleted skin was incapable of initiating a delayed hypersensitivity response to DNCB.[54] Subsequent work with human subjects has shown that LC depletion, determined by either loss of surface marker-positive cells or by ultrastructural criteria, follows single erythemogenic exposures to both sunburn spectrum (UVB) and longwave (UVA) UV light[55-57] and that LC may be reduced in number by 50 to 95% in clinically uninvolved skin of psoriatic patients after several months of psoralen photochemotherapy.[58] Furthermore, unirradiated sun-protected buttock skin of older adult subjects was found to have a nearly 50% reduction ($p = 0.015$) in epidermal LC compared to young adult controls in one study,[56] and habitual sun exposure may further reduce this cell population.[59,60] These combined data suggest that decreased immunologic responsiveness might occur in habitually sun-exposed skin of the elderly as a result of the combined adverse effects on epidermal LC

Table 1
SKIN CANCER IN THE ELDERLY: PROBABLE CONTRIBUTORY FACTORS

Cumulative exposure to carcinogens
Increased induction times
Decreased DNA repair capacity
Decreased immunosurveillance
  (Langerhans cell & T-cell factors)
Decreased melanocytes (UV barrier)
Disturbed regulation of keratinocyte proliferation
Altered dermal matrix

of chronologic aging and repeated UV exposures. Whether a reduction in LC number and/ or function would enhance photocarcinogenesis is unknown. However, the frequent apposition of LC to ''sunburn cells'' within the first hours following UV exposure of human skin and the apparent subsequent migration of these LC from the epidermis suggests that immunologic recognition of UV-altered keratinocytes does occur.[50] The very striking UV-induced systemic immunosuppression elegantly demonstrated by Kripke and co-workers in mice[61-65] may also play a role in human photocarcinogenesis. The possible impact of aging on this phenomenon has not yet been investigated, however.

The role of melanocytes in preventing photocarcinogenesis is incompletely understood. Without question, however, darkly pigmented individuals have a tremendously reduced risk for skin cancer compared to fair-skinned individuals, especially for those lesions most readily attributable to sun exposure;[66,67] and conversely, African[68] and Indian[69] albinos, who presumably differ from other tribe members only in their lack of melanin production, have a much increased risk. It therefore follows that the approximately 50% reduction in dopa-positive (enzymatically active) melanocytes per unit skin surface area which occurs between early and late adulthood in both habitually sun-exposed and sun-protected sites[70-73] should facilitate the development of UV-induced skin cancer in the elderly. Additional studies are needed to determine whether more subtle age-associated defects in melanin production or distribution within the epidermis might further compromise the barrier against UV injury.

Carcinogenesis clearly entails an alteration of cellular growth patterns. The sine qua non of cancer is continued proliferation in the absence of appropriate signals and in abnormal tissue sites. While the acquisition of these abilities is not part of the normal cellular aging process, it is of interest that benign neoplasms are extremely common in old skin[74] and appear to involve all the major cellular and structural elements alone or in combination: keratinocytes, melanocytes, fibroblasts, capillaries, and sebaceous glands.[75,76] Some of these lesions, notably lentigines and sebaceous hyperplasia, occur more frequently in habitually sun-exposed areas; and the premalignant lesions lentigo maligna and actinic keratosis occur almost exclusively in these areas. It seems probable that age-associated loss of proliferative homeostasis at the cellular level[77] — clinically manifested in the skin as acrochordons, seborrheic keratoses, cherry angiomas, lentigines, and other benign growths[74] — compounded by the proliferative and mutagenic effects of UV irradiation[78] increases the likelihood of photocarcinogenesis in the elderly.

A final factor which has been postulated to contribute to the development of skin cancer in habitually irradiated older skin is dermal alteration.[79,79a] Basal cell carcinomas, the most common form of skin cancer,[8] arise almost exclusively in elastotic skin, and it has been suggested that abnormal dermal-epidermal signals promote invagination of basal cell nests into the dermis, resulting in the familiar histologic appearance of these tumors.

VI. PREVENTION AND TREATMENT OF SKIN CANCER IN THE ELDERLY

Nonmelanoma skin cancers are the most common malignancies of man and account for more than 50% of all cancers reported each year in the U.S. Approximately 80% are basal cell carcinomas, and virtually all the remainder are squamous cell carcinomas.[8] Incidences for both forms of skin cancer appear to be increasing in the U.S., approximately 15 to 20% from 1972 to 1978, according to statistics compiled by the National Cancer Institute,[7,8] probably due in part to the increasing proportion of elderly Americans, the group at highest risk, in part to changing lifestyles with increased sun exposure over recent decades, and perhaps in part to depletion of the ozone layer of the earth with the resultant increase in midrange UV intensity of sunlight.[8] For both these reasons, skin cancer ranks as a significant public health problem. Moreover, although cure rates exceed 95% for virtually all treatment modalities in all large series, the actual number of deaths in the U.S. annually ascribed to nonmelanoma skin cancer exceeds that for melanoma,[8] which has itself increased approximately sixfold in incidence over the past 4 decades[80] and is now more common than either Hodgkin's disease or thyroid carcinoma.[81]

The important issues of prevention and treatment of cutaneous malignancy have been the topic of numerous clinical and laboratory studies. It is a sad commentary on the field of dermatologic geriatrics that very few of the existing data have special relevance to the elderly who are the principal patient population for skin cancer. This section attempts to highlight management issues of potential importance in this age group.

A. Prevention

UV irradiation is known to be a major etiologic factor in basal cell carcinoma and squamous cell carcinoma[14,60] and is strongly suspected to contribute to the development of malignant melanoma.[82] Therefore, not surprisingly, prevention of skin cancer is virtually synonymous with sun avoidance. The past decade has witnessed the development and promotion of many highly protective sunscreens[83] capable of blocking 90 to 95% of the "erythemogenic rays,"[83] the enhanced epidermal DNA synthesis[84] that is a presumably necessary intermediary step in oncogenesis,[85] and tumor formation itself in experimental animals.[86]

Recent work with mice emphasizes that these sunscreens also block UV-induced "aging changes"[87] and that the associated histologic changes are partially reversible with time if further UV damage is prevented. However, all human sunscreen trials have utilized young adult volunteers and no study examines the effect of age on sunscreen efficacy by any criteria, either in human skin or in animal skin. This is unfortunate, since diffusion of certain chemicals through the stratum corneum may vary with age and the dose-response curve for at least some clinical, histologic, and biochemical responses in UV-irradiated human skin may be less steep in the elderly than in young adults (see Chapter 2). Since effective sunscreens have only recently become widely available, today's elderly population has certainly not used them for long, and experience with other individually initiated health care options suggests that sunscreens will probably never be used consistently throughout life by the American public, but rather will be used predominantly by middle-aged or elderly people who have already suffered considerable sun damage. Despite these facts, no study has investigated the benefit of beginning sunscreen protection later in life, after tumor initiation has already occurred.

It is well accepted that some squamous cell carcinomas are preceded by distinct premalignant lesions (actinic keratoses on sun-exposed skin or leukoplakia on mucosal surfaces), and anecdotal evidence suggests that individuals with solar keratoses undergo spontaneous regression of these precancerous lesions if excessive sun exposure is discontinued.[88] Quantitative data relating patient age, severity and extent of disease, time required for remission, and the risk of lesional progression to invasive cancer would clearly be of value in managing those older patients for whom excision, cryotherapy, or chemotherapy of premalignant lesions is relatively inconvenient or contraindicated.

Prescription of immunosuppressants or carcinogenic drugs for the elderly is also relevant to cancer prevention in this age group. Experience with renal transplant recipients and other patient groups receiving cyclophosphamide or azothiaprine[89-95] has clearly demonstrated the increased risk of both cutaneous and internal malignancies among those patients on long-term immunosuppressant drugs. In several large series, renal transplant patients have experienced a 2 to 16% incidence of malignancy;[96] among 124 cardiac transplant patients, the actuarial risk of a new cancer was $2.7 \pm 1.9\%$ in the first year and $25.6 \pm 11.0\%$ by 5 years. Overall, 38% of the malignancies reported in immunosuppressed patients occurred in the skin. Most were squamous cell carcinomas, yielding a rate more than 20 times that of the general population, although malignant melanomas were also reported,[96,97] and virtually all tumors occurred in sun-exposed areas.[96] Skin cancer was diagnosed in 8% of all patients within the first year and in 17% of patients following 4 years or longer. Multiple lesions were present in 43% of the patients, and 37 of 521 lesions were known to have metastasized (27 squamous cell carcinomas and 10 melanomas) in one recent review.[96] Patients with successfully treated lymphoreticular malignancies also appear to have an increased incidence of other malignancies as a result of either subtle disease-related immunosuppression or past therapeutic use of carcinogenic agents.[98] While treatment with potentially carcinogenic agents may be necessary for such conditions as Hodgkin's disease and leukemia, it may be optional for patients with mycosis fungoides (cutaneous T-cell lymphoma), for whom several choices of palliative treatments are available.

Because older patients are no longer procreating and because potential induction times for malignancies are short compared to those for young adults, advanced age is often viewed as a relative indication for use of these agents, particularly in situations where they may replace or decrease the requirement for systemic steroids. While this may be a correct posture, the average time to diagnosis of a malignancy in immunosuppressed patients is less than 4 years,[96,99] and as discussed above, older patients appear to have an intrinsically lower threshold for malignancy. At present, there are no data regarding the effect of patient age on the risk of tumor development following treatment with immunosuppressants or directly carcinogenic drugs. Although most reported patients with malignancy following use of immunosuppressant or carcinogenic agents are middle-aged,[96] the population at risk is young, and age-specific data for cancer risk in this population are not available.

B. Treatment

The average American male who was 65 years old in 1980 will live another 14 years; the average woman, more than 18 years.[10] Mean life expectancy at 90 years of age now approaches 5 years in the U.S.[100] Increased physician awareness of this long life expectancy for the elderly has helped to avoid the often disastrous decision not to treat skin cancer on the grounds that death from other causes will supervene before the lesion becomes clinically significant.

Basal cell carcinomas and squamous cell carcinomas are usually treated with one or more of the following: electrosurgery (curettage and electrodesiccation); excision with primary closure, tissue flap rotation, or split-thickness grafting; radiation therapy with external beam or radium implants; liquid nitrogen cryotherapy or microscopically controlled (Mohs') chemosurgery.[101] Cure rates for primary (nonrecurrent) nonmelanoma skin cancer exceed 90% in all large series and approach 100% for small lesions, regardless of treatment modality.[101-104] Approach to a specific lesion is therefore based on multiple criteria including cell type, tumor size and location, cosmesis, patient comfort and convenience, and cost, in addition to anticipated success rate.[101] For elderly patients, general health and mental acuity, presence of specific systemic diseases, ambulatory status, and home environment are frequently important factors in the physician's choice of therapy. Issues directly related to cutaneous aging have not yet been addressed in the literature, but include rate of healing for various types of wounds, character of the resulting scar, intensity of the inflammatory reaction during and after certain procedures, and risk of superinfection.

Premalignant lesions such as actinic keratoses and the much less common keratoacanthoma and lentigo maligna present similar management issues. The decision to treat these lesions at all is complicated by the unknown rate (or indeed risk) of progression to invasive malignancy. For example, although up to 20 to 25% of actinic keratoses are said to eventuate to squamous cell carcinoma,[105,106] the data on which these estimates are based may well suffer from a selection bias, and many dermatologists believe the true figure to be below 1%. Data on lentigo maligna are equally problematic.[108] Hence, the possibility of future malignant conversion must be weighed against the present cost and discomfort of treating these usually asymptomatic lesions. As discussed above, the potential influence of patient age on any of these variables is unknown, and physicians currently must rely on their own experience and biases. Topical 5-fluorouracil appears to be the treatment of choice for widespread actinic keratoses,[109] although light cryotherapy is widely and successfully used for individual lesions.[101] For lentigo maligna, surgical excision probably remains the least controversial form of therapy,[108] although the disadvantages of large facial excisions are obvious. The initial enthusiasm for X-irradiation has been tempered by local recurrence and development of metastatic melanoma in some patients.[110] Recently, argon laser therapy has joined electrosurgery and cryotherapy as alternative treatment modalities.[111]

REFERENCES

1. **Pitot, H. C.,** Carcinogenesis and aging — two related phenomena?, *Am. J. Pathol.,* 87, 44, 1977.
2. **Lundberg, S. and Berge, T.,** Prostatic carcinoma, *Scand. J. Urol. Nephrol.,* 4, 93, 1970.
3. **Berge, T., Ekelund, G., Mellner, C., Phil, B., and Wenckert, A.,** Carcinoma of the colon and rectum in a defined population, *Acta Chir. Scand. Suppl.,* 438, 1973.
4. **Higginson, J. and Muir, C. S.,** *Epidemiology, in Cancer Medicine,* Holland, J. F. and Frei, E., Eds., Lea & Febiger, Philadelphia, 1973.
5. **Ponten, J.,** Abnormal cell growth (neoplasia) and aging, in *Handbook of the Biology of Aging,* Finch, C. E. and Hayflick, L. Eds., Van Nostrand Reinhold Co., New York, 1977, 536.
6. **Scotto, J. and Fears, T. R.,** Skin cancer epidemiology: research needs, *Natl. Cancer Inst. Monogr.,* 50, 169, 1978.
7. **Scotto, J., Kopf, A., and Urbach, F.,** Non-melanoma skin cancer among Caucasians in four areas of the United States, *Cancer,* 34, 1333, 1974.
8. **Scotto, J., Fears, T. R., and Fraumeni, J. F., Jr.,** Incidence of nonmelanoma skin cancer in the United States. U.S. Dept. of Health and Human Services Publication No. (NIH) 82-2433, 1981.
9. **Blum, H. F.,** *Carcinogenesis by Ultraviolet Light,* Princeton University Press, Princeton, N.J., 1979, 340.
9a. **Albert, R. E., Newman, W., and Altshuler, B.,** The dose-response relationships of beta-ray induced skin tumors in the rat, *Radiol. Res.,* 15, 410, 1961.
9b. **Dix, D. and Cohen, P.,** On the role of aging in cancer incidence, *J. Theor. Biol.,* 83, 163, 1980.
10. **Ebbesen, P.,** Aging increases susceptibility of mouse skin to DMBA carcinogenesis independent of general immune status, *Science,* 183, 217, 1974.
11. **Peto, R. F., Roe, J. C., Lee, P. N., Levy, L., and Clark, J.,** Cancer and aging in mice and men, *Br. J. Cancer,* 32, 411, 1975.
12. **Forbes, P. D., Davies, R. E., and Urbach, F.,** Aging, environmental influences, and photocarcinogenesis, *J. Invest. Dermatol.,* 73, 131, 1979.
13. **Smith, K. C.,** Chemical adducts to deoxyribonucleic acid: their importance to the genetic alteration therapy of aging, *Interdiscip. Top. Gerontol.,* 9, 16, 1976.
14. **Culter, R. G.,** Nature of aging and life maintenance processes, *Interdiscip. Top. Gerontol.,* 9, 83, 1976.
15. **Yielding, E. L.,** A model for aging based on differential repair of somatic mutational damage, *Perspect. Biol. Med.,* 17, 210, 1974.

16. **Tice, R. R.,** Aging and DNA-repair capability, in *The Genetics of Aging,* Schneider, E. L., Ed., Plenum Press, New York, 1978, 53.

17. **Hart, R. W. and Setlow, R. B.,** Correlation between deoxyriboncleic acid excision repair and life-span in a number of mammalian species, *Proc. Natl. Acad. Sci. USA,* 71, 2169, 1974.

18. **Lindop, P. J. and Rotblat, J.,** Long-term effects of a single whole-body exposure of mice to ionizing radiations. I. Life-shortening, *Proc. Roy. Soc. (London),* 154, 332, 1961.

19. **Kohn, H. I. and Guttman, P. H.,** Age at exposure and the late effects of X-rays, survival and tumor incidence in CAF mice irradiated at 1 to 2 years of age, *Radiat. Res.,* 18, 348, 1963.

20. **Sacher, G. A.,** Life table modification and life prolongation, in *Handbook of the Biology of Aging,* Finch, C. E. and Hayflick, L., Eds., Van Nostrand Reinhold, New York, 1977, 582.

21. **Martin, G. M.,** Genetic syndromes in man with potential relevance to the pathobiology of aging, in *Genetic Effects of Aging,* Bergsma, D. and Harrison, D. E., Eds, Alan R. Liss for the National Foundation-March of Dimes, New York, 1978.

22. **Holland, J. J., Kohne, D., and Doyle, M. V.,** Analysis of virus replication in aging human fibroblast cultures, *Nature (London),* 245, 316, 1973.

23. **Goldstein, S.,** The role of DNA repair in aging of cultured fibroblasts from xeroderma pigmentosum and normals, *Proc. Soc. Exp. Biol. Med.* 137, 370, 1971.

24. **Painter, R. B., Clarkson, J. M., and Young, B. R.,** Ultraviolet-induced repair replication of aging diploid human cells (WI 38), *Radiat. Res.,* 56, 560, 1973.

25. **Hart, R. W. and Setlow, R. B.,** DNA repair in late passage human cells, *Mech. Aging Dev.,* 5, 67, 1976.

26. **Bowman, P. D., Meek, R. L., and Daniel, C. W.,** Decreased unscheduled DNA synthesis in nondividing aged WI 38 cells, *Mech. Aging Dev.,* 5, 251, 1976.

27. **Cristofalo, V. J. and Sharf, B. B.,** Cellular senescence and DNA synthesis. Thymidine incorporation as a measure of population age in human diploid cells, *Exp. Cell Res.,* 76, 419, 1973.

28. **Epstein, J., Williams, J. R., and Little, J. B.,** Deficient DNA repair in progeria and senescent human cells, *Radiat. Res.,* 55, 527, 1973.

29. **Epstein, J., Williams, J. R., and Little, J. B.,** Rate of DNA repair in progeria and normal human fibroblasts, *Biochem. Biophys. Res. Commun.,* 59, 850, 1974.

30. **Little, J. B., Epstein, J., and Williams, J. R.,** Repair of DNA strand breaks in progeric fibroblasts and aging human diploid cells, in *Molecular Mechanisms for Repair of DNA,* Hanawalt, P. C.and Setlow, R. B., Eds., Plenum Press, New York, 1975, 793.

31. **Mattern, M. R. and Cerutti, P. A.,** Age-dependent excision repair of damaged thymidine from irradiated DNA by isolated nuclei from fibroblasts, *Nature (London),* 254, 450, 1975.

32. **Bender, M. A., Griggs, H. G., and Bedford, J. S.,** Mechanism of chromosomal aberration production. III. Chemicals and ionizing radiation, *Mutat. Res.,* 23, 197, 1974.

33. **Paterson, M. C. Lohman, P. H. M., DeWeerd-Katslein, E. A., and Westerfeld, A.,** Photoreactivation and excison repair of ultraviolet radiation in injured DNA in primary embryonic chick cells, *Biophys. J.,* 14, 454, 1974.

34. **Clarkson, J. M. and Painter, R. B.,** Repair of X-ray damage in aging WI-38 cells, *Mutat. Res.* 23, 107, 1974.

35. **Bradley, M. O., Erickson, L. C., and Kohn, K. W.,** Normal DNA strand rejoining and absence of DNA crosslinking in progeroid and aging human cells, *Mutat. Res.,* 37, 279, 1976.

36. **Little, J. B.,** Relationship between DNA repair capacity and cellular aging, *Gerontology,* 22, 28, 1976.

37. **Sbano, E., Anderassi, L., Fimiani, M., et al.,** DNA-repair after UV-irradiation in skin fibroblasts from patients with actinic keratoses, *Arch. Dermatol.,* 262, 55, 1978.

38. **Lambert, B., Ringborg, V., and Swanbeck, G.,** Ultraviolet-induced DNA repair synthesis in lymphocytes from patients with actinic keratoses, *J. Invest. Dermatol.,* 67, 594, 1976.

39. **Abo-Darub, J. M., Rachie, R., and Pitts, J. D.,** DNA repair deficiency in lymphocytes from patients with actinic keratosis, in *Skin Carcinogenesis,* Pruieras, M., Ed., Masson, Paris, 1978, 357.

40. **Schneider, E. L. and Gilman, B.,** Sister chromatid exchanges and aging. III. The effect of donor age on mutagen-induced sister chromatid exchange in human diploid fibroblasts, *Hum. Genet.,* 46, 57, 1979.

41. **Schneider, E. L. and Monitcone, R. E.,** Aging and sister chromatid exchange. II. The effect of the in vitro passage level of human fetal lung fibroblasts on baseline and mutagen-induced sister chromatid exchange frequencies, *Exp. Cell Res.,* 115, 269, 1978.

42. **Kram, D., Schneider, E. L., Tice, R. R., and Gianas, P.,** Aging and sister chromatid exchange. I. The effect of aging on mitomycin-C induced sister chromatid exchange frequencies in mouse and rat bone marrow cells in vivo, *Exp. Cell Res.,* 114, 471, 1978.

43. **Taichman, L. B. and Setlow, R. B.,** Repair of ultraviolet light damage to the DNA of cultured human epidermal keratinocytes and fibroblasts, *J. Invest. Dermatol.,* 73, 217, 1979.

44. **Hanawalt, P. C., Liu, S. C., and Parsons, C. S.,** DNA repair responses in human skin cells, *J. Invest. Dermatol.,* 77, 86, 1981.

45. **Liu, S. C., Parson, D. S., and Hanawalt, P. C.,** DNA repair response in human epidermal keratinocytes from donors of different age, *J. Invest. Dermatol.,* 79, 330, 1982.

46. **D'Ambrosio, S. M., Slazinski, L., Whetstone, J. W., and Lowney, E.,** Excision repair of UV-induced pyrimidine dimers in human skin in vivo, *J. Invest. Dermatol.,* 77, 311, 1981.

47. **Setlow, R. B.,** Repair deficient human disorders and cancer, *Nature (London),* 271, 713, 1978.

48. **Makinodan, T.,** Immunity and aging, in *Handbook of the Biology of Aging,* Finch, C. E. and Hayflick, L., Eds., Van Nostrand Reinhold Co., New York, 1977, 379.

49. **Burnet, F. M.,** *Immunological Surveillance,* Pergamon Press, Oxford, 1970.

50. **Teller, M. N.,** Age changes and immune resistance to cancer, *Adv. Geront. Res.,* 4, 25, 1972.

51. **Roberts-Thomson, I. C., Whittingham, S., Youngchaiyud, U., et al.,** Aging, immune response, and mortality, *Lancet,* 2, 368, 1974.

52. **Waldorf, D. S., Willkens, R. F., and Decker, J. L.,** Impaired delayed hypersensitivity in an aging population: association with antinuclear reactivity and rheumatoid factor, *JAMA,* 203, 831, 1968.

53. **O'Dell, B. L., Jessen, T., Becker, L. E., Jackson, R. T., and Smith, E. B.,** Diminished immune response in sun-damaged skin, *Arch. Dermatol.,* 116, 559, 1980.

54. **Towes, G. B., Bergstresser, P. R., and Streilein, J. W.,** Epidermal Langerhans cell density determines whether contact hypersensitivity or unresponsiveness follows skin painting with DNFB, *J. Immunol.,* 124, 445, 1980.

55. **Aberer, W., Schuler, G., Stingl, G., Honigsmann, H., and Wolff, K.,** Ultraviolet light depletes surface markers of Langerhans cells, *J. Invest. Dermatol.,* 76, 202, 1981.

56. **Gilchrest, B. A., Murphy, G. F., and Soter, N. A.,** Effect of chronologic aging and ultraviolet irradiation on Langerhans cells in human epidermis, *J. Invest. Dermatol.,* 79, 85, 1982.

57. **Gilchrest, B. A., Soter, N. A., Hawk, J. L. M., Barr, R. M., Black, A. K., Hensby, C. N., Mallet, A. I., Greaves, M. W., and Parrish, J. A.,** Histologic changes associated with UVA-induced erythema in normal human skin, *J. Am. Acad. Dermatol.,* 9, 213, 1983.

58. **Ree, K.,** Reduction of Langerhans cells in human epidermis during PUVA therapy: a morphometric study, *J. Invest. Dermatol.,* 78, 488, 1982.

59. **Delo, V. A., Dawes, L., and Jackson, R.,** Density of Langerhans cells (LC) in normal vs. chronic actinically damaged skin (CADS) of humans, *J. Invest. Dermatol.,* 76, 330, 1981.

60. **Gilchrest, B. A., Szabo, G., Flynn, E., and Goldwyn, R. M.,** Chronologic and actinically-induced aging in human facial skin, *J. Invest Dermatol.,* 80, 81S, 1983.

61. **Kripke, J. L. and Fisher, M. S.,** Immunologic parameters of ultraviolet carcinogenesis, *J. Natl. Cancer Inst.,* 57, 211, 1976.

62. **Fisher, M. S. and Kripke, M. L.,** Systemic alteration induced in mice by ultraviolet light irradiation and its relationship to ultraviolet carcinogenesis, *Proc. Natl. Acad. Sci. USA,* 74, 1688, 1977.

63. **Greene, M. I., Sy, M. S., Kripke, M. L., et al.,** Impairment of antigen-presenting cell function by ultraviolet radiation, *Proc. Natl. Acad. Sci. USA,* 76, 6592, 1979.

64. **Kripke, M. L. and Fidler, I. J.,** Enhanced experimental metastasis of ultraviolet light-induced fibrosarcomas in ultraviolet light-irradiated syngeneic mice, *Cancer Res.,* 40, 625, 1980.

65. **Kripke, M. L.,** Immunologic mechanisms in UV radiation carcinogenesis, *Adv. Cancer Res.,* 34, 69, 1981.

66. **Stoll, H. L., Jr.,** Squamous cell carcinoma, in *Dermatology in General Medicine,* Fitzpatrick, T. B., Eisen, A. Z., Wolff, K., Freedberg, I. M., and Austin, K. F., Eds., McGraw-Hill, New York, 1979, 362.

67. **van Scott, E. J.,** Basal cell carcinoma, in *Dermatology in General Medicine,* Fitzpatrick, T. B., Eisen, A.Z., Wolff, K., Freedberg, I. M., and Austen, K. F., Eds, McGraw-Hill, New York, 1979, 377.

68. **Oettle, A. G.,** Skin cancer in Africa, *Natl. Cancer Inst. Monogr.,* 10, 197, 1963.

69. **Keeler, C. E.,** Albinism, xeroderma pigmentosum, and skin cancer, *Natl. Cancer Inst. Monogr.,* 10, 349, 1963.

70. **Gilchrest, B. A., Blog, F. B., and Szabo, G.,** Effects of aging and chronic sun exposure on melanocytes in human skin, *J. Invest. Dermatol.,* 73, 141, 1979.

71. **Quevedo, W. C., Jr., Szabo, G., and Virks, J.,** Influence of age and UV on the population of dopa-positive melanocytes in human skin, *J. Invest. Dermatol.,* 52, 287, 1969.

72. **Fitzpatrick, T. B., Szabo, G., and Mitchell, R.,** Age changes in the human melanocyte system, in *Advances in the Biology of Skin,* Vol. 6, Montagna, W., Ed., Pergamon Press, Oxford, 1964, 35.

73. **Snell, R. S. and Bischitz, P. G.,** The melanocytes and melanin in human abdominal wall skin: a survey made at different ages in both sexes and during pregnancy, *Ann. Anat. London,* 97, 361, 1963.

74. **Tindall, J. P. and Smith, J. G.,** Skin lesions of the aged, *JAMA,* 186, 1039, 1963.

75. **Gilchrest, B. A.,** Age-associated changes in the skin, *J. Am. Geriatr. Soc.,* 30, 139, 1982.

76. **Lever, W. F. and Schaumberg-Lever, G.,** *Histopathology of the Skin,* J. B. Lippincott Co., Philadelphia, 1975.

77. **Martin, G. M.,** Proliferative homeostasis and its age-related aberrations, *Mech. Aging Dev.,* 9, 385, 1979.

78. **Parrish, J. A., Anderson, R. R., Urbach, F., and Pitts, D.,** *UV-A: Biological Effects of Ultraviolet Radiation with Emphasis on Human Responses to Longwave Ultraviolet,* Plenum Press, New York, 1978.

79. **Getzrow, P. L.,** Histological architecture of basal cell epitheliomas: ectodermal-mesodermal interaction, *Arch Dermatol.,* 94, 44, 1966.

79a. **Pinkus, H.,** The borderline between cancer and noncancer: interrelationships between stroma and epithelium, in *Cancer of the Skin,* Andrade, R., Gumport, S. L, Popkin, G. L., and Rees, T. D., Eds., W. B. Saunders, Philadelphia, 1976, 394.

80. **Elwood, J. A. and Lee, J. A. H.,** Recent data on epidemiology of malignant melanoma, *Semin. Oncol.,* 2, 149, 1975.

81. **Silverberg, E.,** Cancer statistics, 1979, *Cancer,* 29, 6, 1979.

82. **Sober, A. J., Fitzpatrick, T. B., and Mihm, M. C., Jr.,** Primary melanoma of the skin: recognition and management, *J. Am. Acad. Dermatol.,* 2, 179, 1980.

83. **Pathak, M. A.,** Sunscreens: topical and systemic approaches for protective of human skin against harmful effects of solar radiation, *J. Am. Acad. Dermatol.,* 7, 285, 1982.

84. **Lowe, N. J. and Breeding, J.,** Evaluation of sunscreen protection by measurement of epidermal DNA synthesis, *J. Invest. Dermatol.,* 74, 181, 1980.

85. **Epstein, J. H., Fukuyama, K., and Fye, K.,** Effects of ultraviolet radiation on the mitotic cycle and DNA, RNA, and protein synthesis in mammalian epidermis in vivo, *Photchem. Photobiol.,* 12, 57, 1970.

86. **Kligman, L. H., Akin, F., and Kligman, A. M.,** Sunscreens prevent ultraviolet photocarcinogenesis, *J. Am. Acad. Dermatol.,* 3, 30, 1980.

87. **Kligman, L. H., Akin, F. J., and Kligman, A. M.,** Prevention of ultraviolet damage to the dermis of hairless mice by sunscreens, *J. Invest. Dermatol.,* 78, 181, 1982.

88. **Haynes, H. A., Kligman, A. M., and Morison, W.,** Separate personal communications.

89. **Kinlen, L. J., Sheil, A. G. R., Peto, J., and Doll, R.,** Collaborative United Kingdom-Australian study of cancer in patients treated with immunosuppressive drugs, *Br. Med. J.,* 2, 1461, 1969.

90. **Harris, C. C.,** Malignancy during methotrexate and steroid therapy for psoriasis, *Arch. Dermatol.,* 103, 501, 1971.

91. **Penn, I., Haigimson, C. G., and Starzl, T. E.,** De novo malignant tumors in organ transplant recipients, *Transplant. Proc.,* 3, 773, 1971.

92. **Marshall, V. C.,** Premalignant and malignant skin tumours in immunosuppressed patients, *Transplantation,* 17, 272, 1974.

93. **Hill, B. H. R.,** Immunosuppressive drug therapy as a potentiator of skin tumours in five patients with lymphoma, *Aust. J. Dermatol.,* 17, 46, 1976.

94. **Arseneau, J. C., Canellos, G. P., Johnson, R., and DeVita, V. T.,** Risk of new cancers in patients with Hodgkin's disease, *Cancer,* 40, 1912, 1977.

95. **Maize, J. C.,** Skin cancer in immunosuppressed patients, *JAMA,* 237, 1857, 1977.

96. **Penn, I.,** The price of immunotherapy, *Curr. Probl. Surg.,* 18, 681, 1981.

97. **Chaudhuri, P. K., Walker, M. J., and Das Gupta, T. K.,** Cutaneous malignant melanoma after immunosuppressive therapy, *Arch. Surg.,* 115, 322, 1980.

98. **Lee, L. A., Fritz, K. A., Golitz, L., Fritz, T, J., and Weston, W. L.,** Second cutaneous malignancies in patients with mycosis fungoides treated with topical nitrogen mustard, *J. Am. Acad. Dermatol.,* 7, 590, 1982.

99. **Harrington, W. J.,** Iatrogenic disorders from cancer treatment, *Adv. Int. Med.,* 24, 141, 1979.

100. Health Care Financing Administration, Discussion Paper: Long-Term Care: Background and Future Directions, U.S. Government Publication No. (HFCA) 81-20047, 1981.

101. **Albright, S D., III,** Treatment of skin cancer using multiple modalities, *J. Am. Acad. Dermatol.,* 7, 143, 1982.

102. **Freeman, R. G., Knox, J. M., and Heaton, C. L.,** Treatment of skin cancer: statistical study of 1,341 skin tumors comparing results obtained with irradiation, surgery, and curettage followed by electrodesiccation, *Cancer,* 17, 535, 1964.

103. **Chernovsky, M. E.,** Squamous cell and basal cell carcinomas: preliminary study of 3,817 primary skin cancers, *South. Med. J.,* 71, 802, 1978.

104. **Mohs, F. E.,** Chemosurgery for the microscopically controlled excision of cutaneous cancer, in *Skin Surgery,* 4th ed., Epstein, E. and Epstein, E., Jr., Eds., Charles C Thomas, Springfield, Ill., 1977, 526.

105. **Montgomery, H.,** Precancerous dermatosis and epithelioma in situ, *Arch. Dermatol.,* 39, 387, 1939.

106. **Caro, W. A.,** Tumors of the skin, in *Dermatology,* Moschella, S. L., et al., Eds., W. B. Saunders, Philadelphia, 1975, 1323.

107. **Pinkus, H.,** Actinic keratosis—actinic skin, in *Cancer of the Skin,* Andrade, R., Gumport, S. L., Popkin, G. L., Rees, T. D., Eds., W. B. Saunders, Philadelphia, 1976, 437.

108. **Goette, D. K.,** Topical chemotherapy of solar keratoses, *Med. J. Aust.,* 2, 1136, 1969.

109. **Sober, A. J., Mihm, M. C., Jr., Fitzpatrick, T. B., and Clark, W. H., Jr.,** Malignant melanoma of the skin, and benign neoplasms and hyperplasias of melanocytes in the skin, in *Dermatology in General Medicine,* McGraw-Hill, New York, 1979, 629.

110. **Kopf, A. W., Bart, R. S., and Gladstein, A. H.,** Treatment of melanotic freckle with X-rays, *Arch. Dermatol.,* 112, 801, 1976.

111. **Arndt, K. A.,** Argon laser therapy of lentigo maligna, *J. Am. Acad. Dermatol.,* in press.

Chapter 7

IN VITRO STUDIES OF AGING IN THE SKIN

I. INTRODUCTION

Aging was among the first problems to be studied in tissue culture. Alexis Carrel, a renowned biologist working at the Rockefeller Institute for Medical Research in the early 1900s, published in 1911 the first method for cultivation of epithelial or fibroblast cells from explant fragments of normal and malignant mammalian tissues.[1] The following year he published a modification of the method which prolonged survival of the cultures from a maximum of 20 days to more than 3 months, and at this time postulated that somatic cells would not age in vitro, but would be found to have a "permanent life," once adequate culture conditions were developed.[2] In 1913, Carrel reported that some chicken embryo cell strains had been maintained in continuous culture for more than 16 months and 190 serial passages and referenced the previous paper as demonstration that "connective tissue cells can be preserved permanently in vitro in a condition of active life."[3] Using this culture system, Carrel performed a series of then-elegant gerontologic experiments. He first demonstrated that plasma (the major component of his culture medium) obtained from 4 to 5-month-old chickens supported faster growth of fibroblasts than did plasma from 4 to 5-year-old chickens and suggested that the ability of plasma to support culture growth could be used as a quantitative marker of physiologic age for the organism, the first of many proposed "aging indices." He then cultured tissues from chick embryos and young and old adult chickens in adult chicken plasma and demonstrated that "the velocity of growth always varied in inverse ratio to the age of the animal from which the tissue has been extirpated."[3] In his final publication addressing the question of senescence in vitro,[4] Carrel reported experiments in which chick fibroblasts from a "strain" already carried 9 years in continuous culture were transferred to paired dishes containing plasma from chickens aged 6 weeks, 3 months, 3 years, or 9 years. In all instances, there was an inverse relationship between age of the plasma donor and both rate of multiplication and in vitro life span for the chick fibroblasts (Figures 1 and 2). Further experiments suggested that these results were more consistent with an age-related increase in a serum inhibitor of growth than with a decrease in a serum promotor of growth (Figure 3), a hypothesis still under investigation.[5] Unfortunately for the field of gerontology, neither Carrel nor later investigators noted the contradiction between the "permanent life" of the fibroblasts used in these experiments and their finite life span (never more than 23 passages) after beginning the experiments. In retrospect, Carrel's "permanent" strains were probably the result of repeated inoculation of his cultures with fresh fetal fibroblasts present as contaminants in the "embryo extract" used to supplement the plasma- and serum-based media fed to the cultures at 2 to 3-day intervals.[2] (During the aging experiments, embryo extract was omitted from the media.[4]) In any case, Carrel's conclusion[2-4] that individual somatic cells were immortal and that aging resulted from changes in the plasma (or other extracellular compartment) foreclosed the field of cellular aging for half a century. His own fibroblast line was voluntarily terminated after 34 years[6] and the observation of "permanent life" was confirmed over the ensuing decades by many investigators who established immortal cell lines from a variety of tissues and species, using progressively more sophisticated techniques. (These cells have since been found to be karyotypically abnormal, spontaneously or virally transformed lines.) When later investigators reported finite life spans for cultured cells, their results were attributed to inadequate culture conditions.

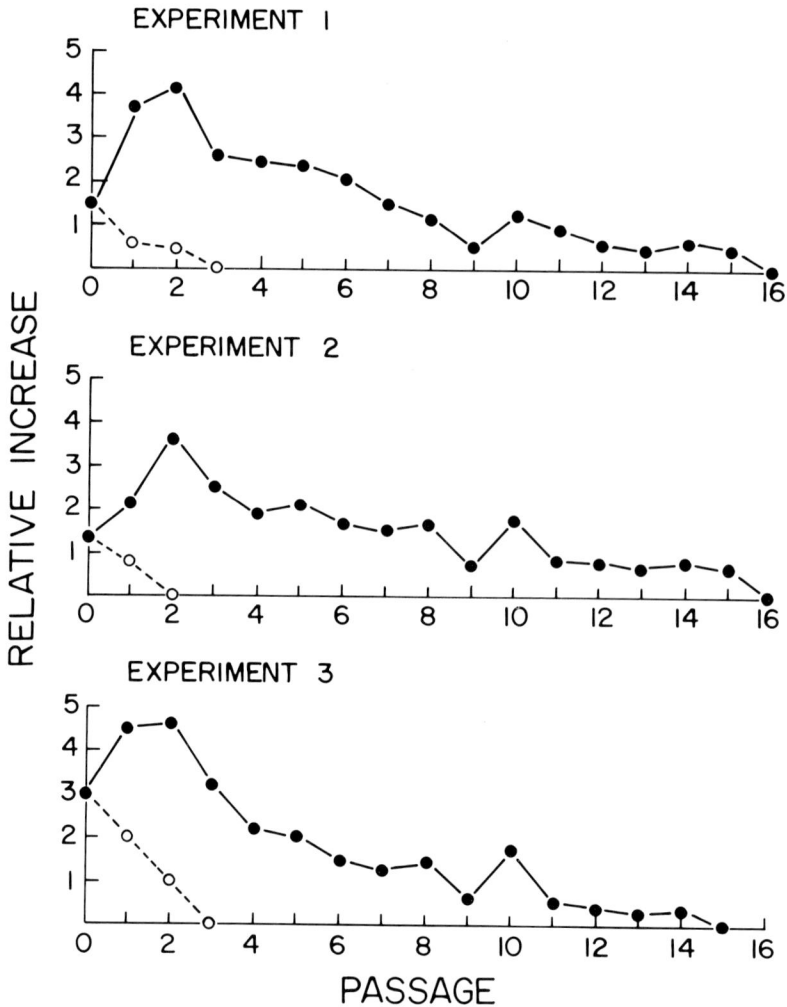

FIGURE 1. Relationship between rate of cellular growth and age of the plasma donor. Chick fibroblasts were grown using early tissue culture methodology in the presence of plasma derived from chickens of various age. Data from three separate experiments comparing 3-month-old chick plasma (●) to 9-year-old cock plasma (○) are shown. Growth is much faster and continues longer in the younger plasma. (Modified and reproduced from Carrel, A. and Ebeling, A. H., *J. Exp. Med.*, 34, 599, 1921, by copyright permission of the Rockefeller University Press.)

II. IN VITRO FIBROBLAST AGING (HAYFLICK MODEL)

In vitro aging research was reborn in 1961, when Hayflick and Moorehead[7] reported that cultured human fetal lung fibroblasts underwent a finite reproducible number of serial passages or cumulative population doublings (CPD). Furthermore, fetal fibroblasts were capable of 35 to 63 CPD under the conditions employed, while adult-derived fibroblasts were capable of only 14 to 39 CPD.[8] Hayflick's interpretation of this phenomenon as aging at the cellular level, analogous to and perhaps underlying aging of the intact organism[8-10] created an in vitro fibroblast model of aging.

Fetal lung fibroblast strains (initially WI-38 and more recently also IMR-90 and others), frozen in large numbers at early passage and made readily available to interested scientists, have since been used extensively for gerontologic studies. The model equates fetal cells at early passage with "youth" and those at late passage, just prior to total loss of proliferative capacity, with "old age."

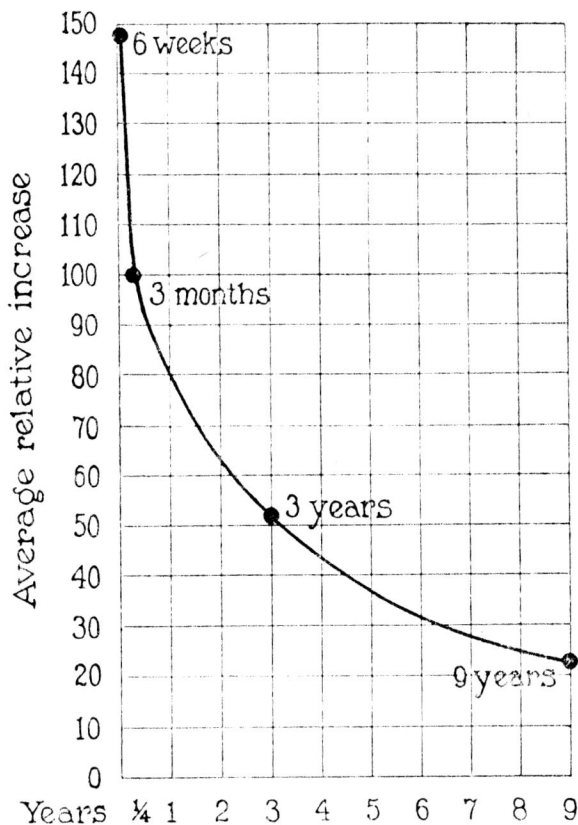

FIGURE 2. Summary graph comparing rates of fibroblast growth in chicken plasma from donors aged 6 weeks, 3 months, 3 years, and 9 years. Identical relationships were obtained for culture life span vs. plasma donor age. (Reproduced from Carrel, A. and Ebeling, A. H., *J. Exp. Med.*, 34, 599, 1921, by copyright permission of the Rockefeller University Press.)

Further evidence that the proliferative limit for cultured cells in some way corresponds to aging in vivo includes: (1) Grafts of mammary tissue, skin, and bone marrow serially transplanted to young isogenic hosts eventually senesce and die, and graft survival time may be inversely proportional to the age of the original tissue donor,[10,11] although interpretation is difficult in many experiments. (2) Culture life span of embryonic fibroblasts is inversely related (with some exceptions[12]) to the maximum life span of the donor species.[11] (3) Human dermal fibroblast life span in vitro is inversely proportional to donor age in healthy adult populations,[13,14] decreasing a calculated 0.2 CPD per year of donor age,[13] and is shortened, relative to age-matched controls in subjects with progeria,[13,15] Werner's syndrome[13] and even diabetes,[13,16,17] disorders believed by many authorities to represent premature aging. The more recent emphasis on dermal fibroblasts from young vs. old adult donors, rather than early vs. late passage fetal lung fibroblasts, reflects the concern that the former comparison may be more relevant to aging in vivo. This concern has been given experimental support by the demonstration that cultured fibroblasts from young and old adults differ in ways qualitatively and quantitatively dissimilar from early vs. late passage WI-38 cells.[14]

Although the inverse relationship between donor age and cultured fibroblast life span is well documented, the mechanism of this eventual proliferative failure is unknown. Present evidence fails to implicate faulty DNA repair, replication, or transcription; protein synthesis; or intermediary metabolism.[10] Recent work has suggested that inability to respond to ap-

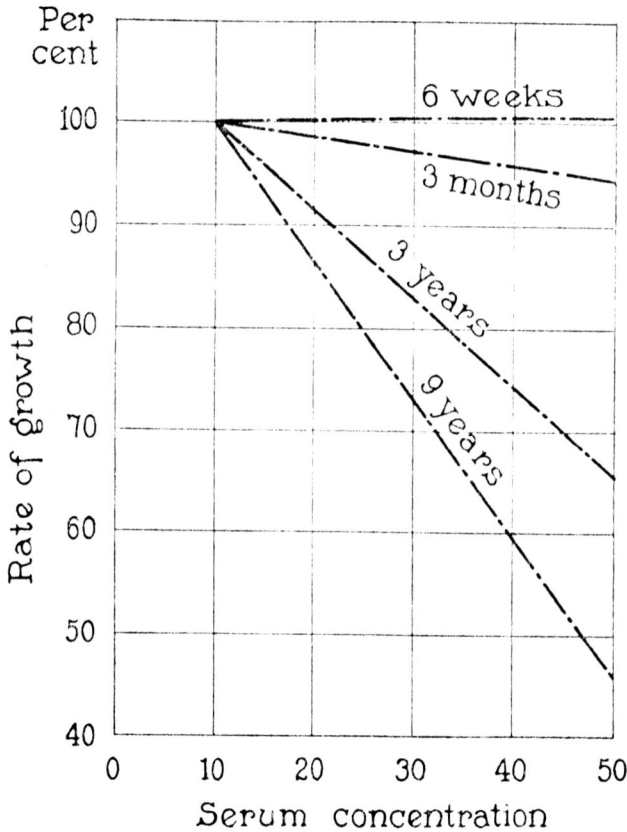

FIGURE 3.   Evidence for an age-associated plasma inhibitor of cellular growth. Rate of growth (relative to that obtained in culture medium containing 10% serum) is shown for chick fibroblasts maintained in different concentrations of serum derived from chickens aged 6 weeks, 3 months, 3 years, and 9 years. Progressively less growth is achieved with all but the youngest serum batch at higher concentrations, suggesting the presence of an inhibitor which accumulates or becomes more effective with increasing donor age. As indicated in Figures 1 and 2, older sera also supported less rapid growth in the baseline 10% concentration than did younger sera. (Reproduced from Carrel, A. and Ebeling, A. H., *J. Exp. Med.*, 34, 599, 1921, by copyright permission of the Rockefeller University Press.)

propriate mitogens in the cell's environment may be responsible in part. With increasing passage level in vitro, WI-38 fibroblasts have been shown to require a higher concentration of dialyzed fetal serum to obtain a given proliferative rate (one population doubling in 4 days), and total culture growth prior to senescence increases with increasing maintenance concentrations of fetal serum from early passage.[20] The same fibroblast strain shows a diminished proliferative response to hydrocortisone and has fewer specific binding sites per cell at late passage.[21,22] Harley et al.[22a] have reported that the concentrations of an insulin-like preparation necessary to stimulate 50 and 95% maximal DNA synthesis in dermal fibroblast cultures are greater for late passage than for early passage cells and greater at early passage for cells derived from three donors aged 67 to 76 years than for cells derived from three donors aged 22 to 24 years. Finally, early passage dermal fibroblasts derived from adult truncal skin display decreased responsiveness to serum mitogens and to insulin, thrombin, and epidermal growth factor in serum-free medium, compared to those derived from newborn foreskin.[22c] Similarly, adult dermal fibroblasts have been reported to require 10-fold more platelet-derived growth factor than do fetal fibroblasts for optimal growth,[22b] although the use of possibly senescent adult cells in these experiments complicates interpretation of the data.

Table 1
SKIN CANCER IN THE ELDERLY:
PROBABLE CONTRIBUTORY
FACTORS

Cumulative exposure to carcinogens
Increased induction times
Decreased DNA repair capacity
Decreased immunosurveillance
 (Langerhans cell & T-cell factors)
Decreased melanocytes (UV barrier)
Disturbed regulation of keratinocyte proliferation
Altered dermal matrix

Age-related changes in metabolic as well as proliferative hormonal responses have been studied using cultured human dermal fibroblasts. Harley, Goldstein, and co-workers measured stimulation of glucose uptake and DNA synthesis by a human plasma derived preparation with insulin-like activity (ILA) in both early and late passage fibroblasts from four young (22 to 28 years old) and four old (67 to 76 years old) adults, from a 9-year-old progeric patient and two age-matched controls.[22a] Early passage cells from old donors (and the progeric patient) required a two- to threefold higher ILA concentration than did cells from young donors to achieve equivalent stimulation of DNA synthesis ($p < 0.01$), but donor age did not affect ILA-stimulated glucose uptake. The authors suggest that ILA may exert its metabolic and proliferative effects via different receptors, and that only the receptor mediating DNA synthesis is affected by aging. Other differences in fibroblast responsiveness to ILA were related to passage level or the progeric state and serve to emphasize the discrepancies between in vivo aging, in vitro aging, and pathologic "premature" aging.

In addition to proliferative potential and metabolic responsiveness, numerous morphologic, biochemical, and physiologic parameters have been studied as a function of age in cultured fibroblasts.[10,18,19] No clear concensus regarding the cause(s) of aging has yet emerged, but the now extensive data form an excellent foundation for future, more directed inquiries.

Despite the limitations of these fibroblast models, the apparent correspondence between chronologic or physiologic age and the life span of cultured cells provides an opportunity to investigate the basis of aging at the cellular level (rather than in the more complex intact organism), an in vitro means of assessing tissue age, and the theoretic possibility of quantifying adverse or beneficial environmental influences on the intrinsic aging process.

III. IN VITRO KERATINOCYTE AGING

The development in 1975 of a method for serial cultivation of disaggregated human keratinocytes at low density[23] greatly expanded opportunities for in vitro investigation of this cell type and provided an ideal opportunity to study aging in a differentiating cell type. Although the keratinocyte's specialized functions such as keratin protein production and barrier formation have not yet been explored in a gerontologic context, several studies have examined the age-associated loss of keratinocyte proliferative potential.

In their original publication,[23] Rheinwald and Green compared the in vitro proliferative behavior of seven newborn-derived keratinocyte cultures to that of three cultures derived from donors age 3, 12, and 34 years. Newborn cultures underwent a calculated 25 to 31 cell generations and could be maintained through 3 to 6 passages, while the older cultures underwent 20 to 27 generations and could be maintained through only 2 to 3 passaged under identical conditions. Plating efficiency (visible colonies per 100 cells inoculated) ranged up to 15.7% for the newborn keratinocytes and usually exceeding 2%, while the highest plating efficiency observed for the post-newborn keratinocytes was 0.7% for the 12-year donor.

Total keratinocyte population expansion in culture averaged 5737-fold for the newborn keratinocytes and exceeded 100,000-fold for two of these donors, while population expansion averaged 333-fold for the three older donors, and was 2.6-fold for the only adult donor. These data strongly suggested that donor age influences keratinocyte life span and proliferative capacity in vitro and that quantitative effects are comparable to those observed for dermal fibroblasts.

The same laboratory has demonstrated that culture life span for the keratinocyte is dependent on the presence or absence of certain well-defined growth promoting factors: hydrocortisone, epidermal growth factor (EGF), and cholera toxin.[24] The observed influence of hydrocortisone was subtle and manifested only in post-primary cultures as the continued formation of colonies with small actively multiplying basal keratinocytes, in contrast to the earlier loss of such colonies in cultures lacking the steroid.[23,24] The beneficial effect of EGF could be detected earlier, at a time when individual colonies contained 50 to 200 cells (approximately 6 to 8 cell generations), although not earlier, and was manifested as reduced stratification of colonies with a subsequently larger basal population, a prolongation of the period of rapid cell division in serially passaged cultures, and an increased plating efficiency in post-primary cultures.[24,25] These effects increased the calculated culture life span for newborn keratinocytes from approximately 50 to 150 cell generations[25] and were especially noticeable at late passage, when keratinocytes grown in the absence of EGF were "senescent." Cholera toxin, the most effective of several agents known to increase intracellular cAMP,[26] had the most striking effect on culture life span and growth rate of the factors studied in this system.[24] The effect of cholera toxin on keratinocyte growth could be detected within the first week of culture and was manifested by a decrease in the calculated cell doubling time, an apparent increase in the calculated total generations in vitro and in the number of serial passages obtained.[24,26] These effects were also reported to be much more prominent in keratinocyte cultures derived from adults than from newborns, and at late passage than at early passage.[24]

Keratinocyte cultures have also been utilized to assess in vitro physiologic age.[27,28] Keratinocytes derived from paired skin biopsies of the lateral (sun-exposed) and medial (nonexposed) aspects of the upper arm in adult donors were maintained under identical conditions in the Rheinwald-Green system and serially passaged until senescence. In all instances, total generations in culture were less for the cultures derived from sun-exposed skin, and the discrepancy in culture life span between cultures from the two sites increased linearly with donor age and clinical evidence of sun-induced "premature aging".[27] Similar reductions in the life span of dermal fibroblasts attributable to chronic sun exposure were measured in the same skin specimens,[29] further emphasizing the comparability of keratinocytes and fibroblasts for in vitro studies of aging. Absolute values for keratinocyte generations were comparable to those reported by Rheinwald and Green,[23] although no consistent relationship between donor age and culture life span was apparent. Confirmatory keratinocyte data were obtained in a parallel study utilizing paired pre-auricular (sun-exposed) and post-auricular (nonexposed) facial skin[28] (see also Chapter 8).

Systematic studies of cultured keratinocytes designed to assess histologic changes as a function of donor age have not been reported. The fact that epidermal keratinocytes in vivo manifest only very slight organizational or ultrastructural changes with age[30] suggests that this may not be a rewarding approach, although subtle abnormalities of stratified colony morphology may distinguish adult from newborn cultures.[28] In vitro keratinocyte aging (late passage vs. early passage, regardless of donor age) appears to include the appearance of irregular colonies composed primarily of large keratincoytes in contrast to the nearly round colonies composed of uniformly small cells that characterize primary cultures.[24] At late passage, small colonies may manifest greater stratification than at early passage: large colonies contain 5 to 7 cell layers centrally in this system regardless of passage level.[28] At

A

FIGURE 4.   Electron micrographs of keratinocyte colonies derived from the preauricular skin specimen of a 55-year-old woman. (A) Primary culture nearing confluence. Note close apposition of the keratinocyte membranes with frequent desmosomes and normal-appearing subcellular organelles. Boundaries between cells (*) allow identification of 6 cell layers. (B) Tertiary culture at senescence. Note keratinocytes undergoing autolysis (A) with loss of organelles. Intercellular boundaries (arrowheads) even between morphologically normal keratinocytes lack desmosomes; in many areas intercellular spaces are widened. (Scale bar = 1 μ, original magnification 12,000×. Reproduced with permission from Gilchrest, B. A., et al., *J. Invest. Dermatol.*, 80, 81S, 1983.)

the ultrastructural level keratinocyte colonies at late passage are characterized by larger intracellular spaces, fewer desmosomes, and more frequent intracellular vacuoles than are equally large early passage cultures from the same donor[28] (Figure 4). The causal relationship, if any, of these changes to keratinocyte senescence is unknown.

DNA replication and repair capacity have recently been examined in keratinocyte cultures derived from newborn vs. adult skin. In studies using a culture system that supports modest net growth for approximately 2 weeks and some keratinocyte survival for at least 1 month, cell survival is reduced and semiconservative DNA replication over 24 hr is inhibited to an equal extent in both newborn and adult cultures by UV (254 nm) radiation.[30a] DNA repair over the ensuing 24 hr, assayed by the 5-bromodeoxyuridine (5-BrUdR) density labeling method, follows a similar time course and a similar dose-response curve with increasing UV exposure in both groups.[30a] Absolute values for 5-BrUdR labeling were not specified, but keratinocyte excision repair in vitro has been reported in previous studies to be comparable to that of dermal fibroblasts.[30b,30c] However, as noted by the authors, DNA repair rates for human skin in vivo are more rapid,[30d] suggesting that repair may be compromised in this culture system.

In vitro assessment of certain aspects of keratinocyte behavior has been facilitated by the recent development of culture systems that are independent of serum and co-cultivated

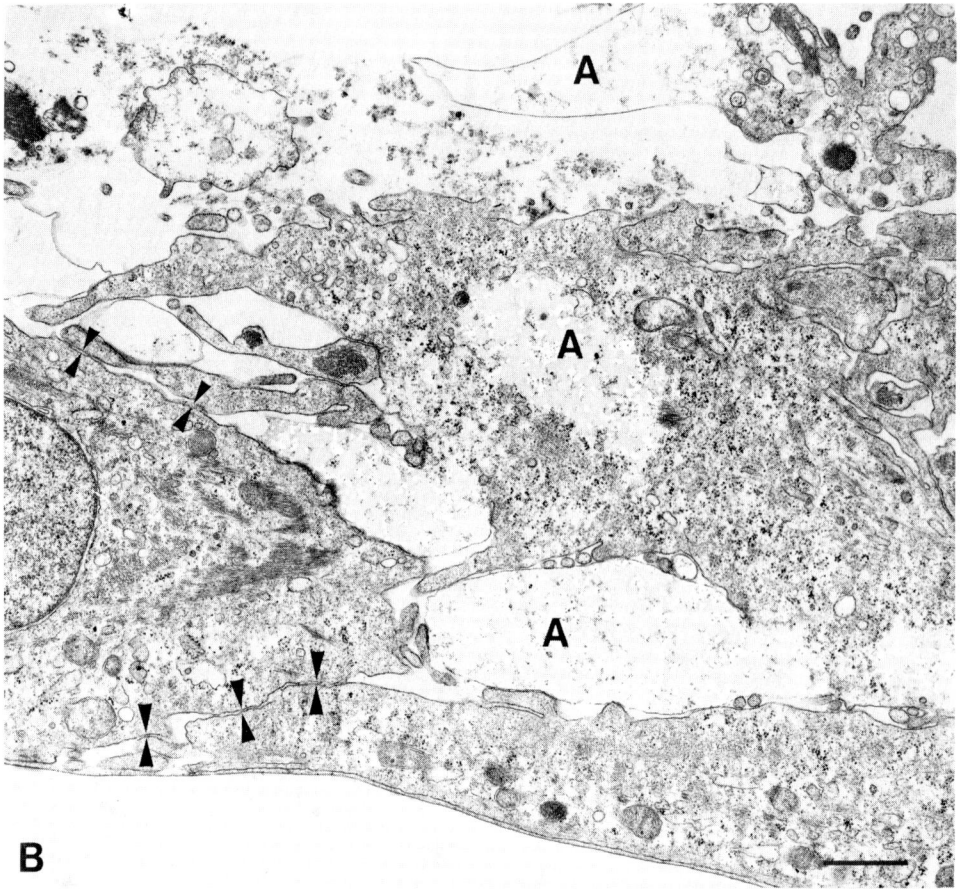

FIGURE 4B

fibroblast-like cells. Such a system has recently been used to investigate the possible influence of donor age on the growth factor responsiveness of human keratinocytes in vitro.[31] These experiments address the hypothesis mentioned above that in vitro senescence, the ultimate failure of cells to proliferate in an environment which initially supported exponential growth, may result from an acquired inability to respond to specific growth factors in the medium.[20,21] Attachment rate for keratinocytes derived from four newborns and four adults aged 26 to 62 years varied from 25 to 40% with no differences between the groups, but newborn cells grew better than adult cells plated at equal density under identical conditions, and manifested steeper dose-response curves to selected mitogens in this system[31] (Figures 5 and 6).

It must be noted that comparisons between newborns and adults incorporate the methodologic error of comparing *developing* and *mature* tissue rather than *young* mature and *old* mature tissues. Such comparisons are of value, however, in identifying trends that may indeed be relevant to the aging process but are too subtle to detect in small studies of exclusively adult tissue with current techniques.

IV. IN VITRO DISCREPANCIES BETWEEN KERATINOCYTES AND FIBROBLASTS RELEVANT TO AGING STUDIES

The rather striking analogies in vitro between aging keratinocytes and fibroblasts should not obscure the important behavioral differences of these two cell types.

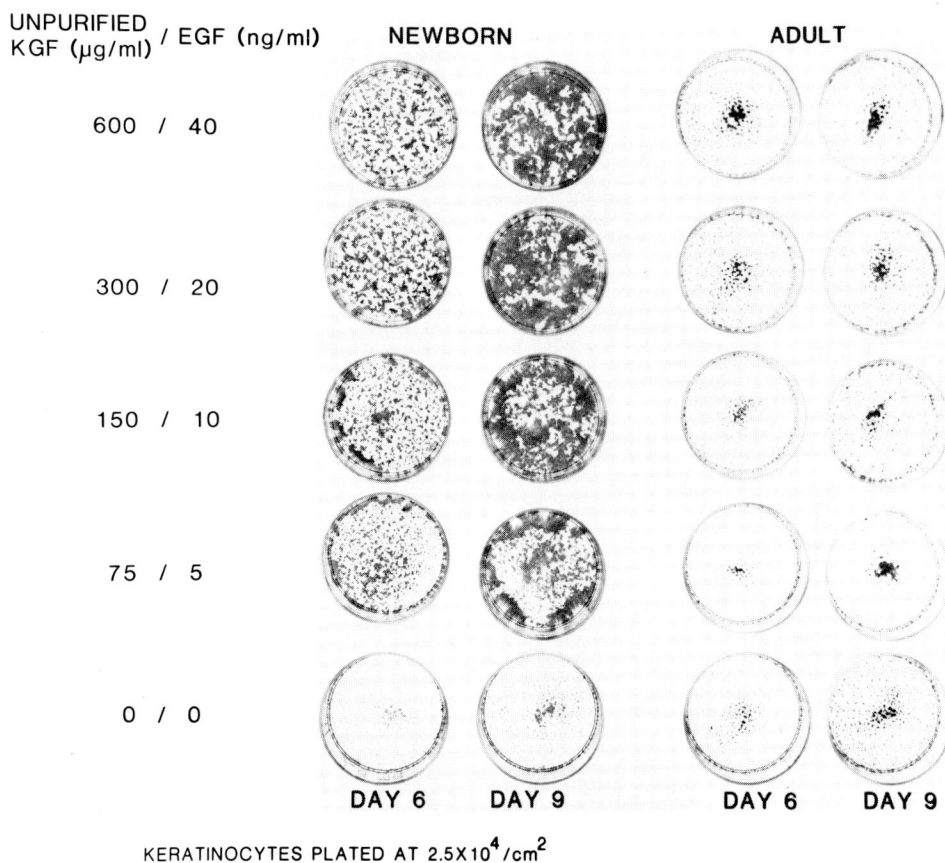

UNPURIFIED KGF (µg/ml) / EGF (ng/ml)	NEWBORN	ADULT
600 / 40		
300 / 20		
150 / 10		
75 / 5		
0 / 0		
	DAY 6 DAY 9	DAY 6 DAY 9

KERATINOCYTES PLATED AT $2.5 \times 10^4/cm^2$

FIGURE 5.   Effect of donor age on growth factor responsiveness of human keratinocytes in vitro. Keratinocytes from single near-confluent primary cultures derived from either newborn foreskin or truncal skin of a healthy 62-year-old adult were replated at 2.5×10^4 cell/cm² on dishes coated with human fibronectin 10 µg/cm² in M199 (GIBCO) supplemented with hydrocortisone $1.4 \times 10^{-6}M$, insulin 10 µg/mℓ, transferrin 10 µg/mℓ, triiodothyronine $10^{-9}M$, bovine serum albumin 2 mg/mℓ, and the indicated concentrations of epidermal growth factor (EGF) and a bovine hypothalamic extract known to contain a potent mitogen, keratinocyte growth factor (KGF). Cultures were maintained in their respective media, re-fed at 3-day intervals, and duplicate plates were stained after 6 days or 9 days with Rhodanile blue. Newborn cultures showed strikingly better growth overall than adult cultures and a greater response to EGF and KGF. Experiments using EGF and KGF individually gave similar results. Plates shown are representative of those from four newborn and four adult donors. (Reproduced with permission from Gilchrest, B. A., *J. Invest. Dermatol.*, 81, 184S, 1983.

Central to the in vitro model of cellular aging is the observation that culture life span, reported as "cumulative population doublings," is inversely proportional to the age of the tissue donor. CPD is equivalent to total cell generations if one assumes all cells in the original population undergo mitosis, all have the same cell cycle time, and all daughter cells join the proliferative compartment. Although clearly not quite correct for the fibroblast,[32-35] these assumptions still allow collection of meaningful data. In the case of cultured keratinocytes, these assumptions are very far from true: rarely do 10% of plated cells successfully establish colonies under optimal conditions, and the fraction is more often well below 1%.[23,26] In addition, a variable portion of daughter cells leave the basal layer of the colonies, "terminally differentiate," and cease to proliferate. Even in the basal layer, not all keratinocytes in rapidly growing large colonies incorporate thymidine during a 24-hr period,[23,37] although it is not known whether these cells could resume mitotic cycling if appropriately stimulated.

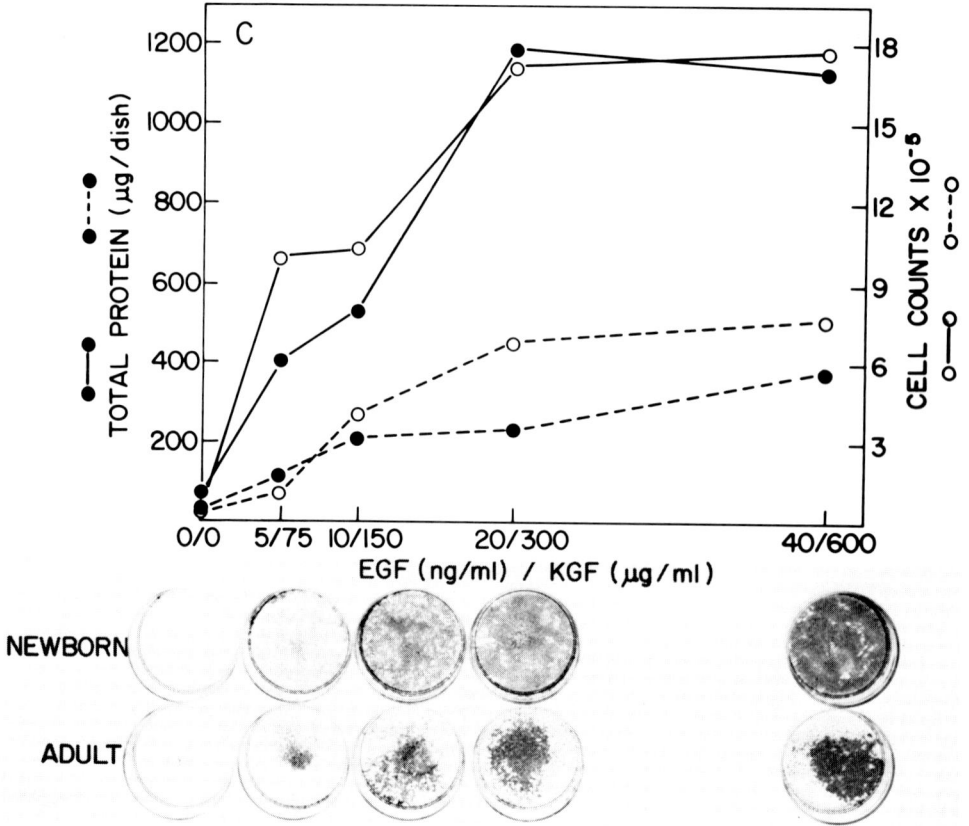

FIGURE 6.   Quantitative assessment of keratinocyte responsiveness to specific mitogens as a function of donor age. Single primary keratinocyte culture dishes derived from a newborn ●–○ and a 20-year-old adult ○--○ donor were passaged at $10^4/cm^2$ and maintained as specified in Figure 5. After 7 days, paired plates were fixed and stained with Rhodanile blue, counted in a hemocytometer chamber, or assayed for total protein content. EGF/KGF concentrations varied from 0/0 to 40 ng/mℓ / 600 µg/mℓ (4 × standard medium concentrations). Each point graphed is the mean of 2 or 3 determinations from a single plate. Excellent concordance for cell number, total protein, and colony size is apparent. Growth of newborn keratinocytes is superior to that of adult keratinocytes in all media tested. In addition, the dose-response curves are steeper for the newborn than for the adult cultures. (Reproduced with permission from Gilchrest, B. A., *J. Invest. Dermatol.* 81, 184S, 1983.)

For all these reasons, other means of estimating total cell generations for cultured kera-tinocytes must be employed. One possible approach for experiments conducted in the Rhein-wald-Green system[23] is to use the following definitions and assumptions:[27] plating efficiency: the number of epidermal colonies visible on a stained plate after 3 weeks growth, divided by the total number of cells originally plated. Average number of cells per colony (CPC): after removing fibroblasts from the plate, the remaining cells (keratinocytes) are trypsinized and counted, and this number is divided by the number of colonies on paired stained plates. Number of keratinocyte generations per passage (G):2^G = number of cells created by a single progenitor after G generations, i.e., the number of CPD. G = ln(CPC)/ln2. At low plating density, it is safe to assume that all colonies arise from single cells, but this calculation also assumes that every cell capable of establishing a visible colony and all its progeny subsequently continue to divide at the same rate as all other colony-forming cells on the plate. Perhaps surprisingly, total keratinocyte generations calculated in this way closely conform to total fibroblast generations calculated as CPD for same age donor, roughly 25 to 50 for cells derived from newborn skin, and 10 to 20 for cells derived from adult skin.[23,27,28]

Attachment rate (percent cells adherent at 2 to 24 hr) and plating efficiency (percent cells forming visible colonies, i.e., undergoing at least four population doublings after 2 to 4 weeks) are comparable and usually exceed 90% in fibroblast cultures,[14,23] while these figures are quite dissimilar for keratinocyte cultures. Keratinocytes attachment rate averages approximately 30 to 35% under current optimal conditions[31,36] and is independent of donor age;[31] while plating efficiency, which must at present be determined in different culture systems, is roughly 1 to 10% in newborn cultures[23] and frequently below 0.01% in adult cultures.[23,27]

V. IN VITRO STUDIES OF OTHER CUTANEOUS CELLS

The skin contains at least seven cell types amenable to in vitro aging studies. In addition to keratinocytes and fibroblasts, there are melanocytes, Langerhans cells, microvascular endothelial cells, and adipocytes, spanning a broad spectrum of embryologic origins and biologic functions. Rapidly evolving culture techniques should soon permit meaningful gerontologic studies in vitro.

Recently developed systems for human melanocytes already permit survival of virtually pure newborn cultures for up to 21 CPD and 32 weeks in the presence of phorbol ester[38] and up to 10 CPD and 4 weeks in its absence.[39] Preliminary studies with these systems suggest that melanocytes derived from adult skin have a considerably shorter average life span in vitro and decreased response to specific mitogens.

Although identification and partial isolation of endothelial cells in vitro has been reported by many investigators over the past decade, only recently have long-term cultures been achieved,[40-42] opening the door to in vitro gerontologic investigation of endothelial cells derived from the dermal microvasculature. As with keratinocytes, microvascular endothelial cells derived from newborn foreskin have been utilized by most investigators,[41,43] presumably because of greater proliferative capacity, although adult tissue is adequate is some systems.[40,44] In long-term cultures, endothelial cell life span is strongly dependent on the hormonal environment,[42,45] again in a manner analogous to the epidermal keratinocyte.[24] Gerontologic studies of cultured endothelial cells from the microvasculature have not yet been reported, but large vessel endothelial cells have already been used to corroborate earlier fibroblast findings.[42,45,46]

VI. RELEVANCE TO IN VIVO AGING

The relevance of the in vitro findings discussed above to the aging process in man or other animals is unclear and may be nonexistent. It has been observed that tissues serially passaged in syngeneic hosts have a life span exceeding that of the donor animal, and that organisms rarely if ever die because of lost cellular proliferative capacity. The possibly unique example of a cell population frequently exhausted during the human life span is hair bulb melanocytes. These cells, called upon to proliferate extensively during each anagen cycle of hair growth, frequently disappear from the follicle beginning in the fourth or fifth decade.[47] "Greying," or more correctly progressive replacement of pigmented hairs by white ones, first occurs on the scalp where the ratio of anagen (growth) to telogen (resting) phase is greater than at other body sites, and melanocyte "senescence" might therefore be expected to occur first. A second potential example of this phenomenon is the late bone marrow failure occasionally seen in X-irradiated patients and experimental animals. After recovering from the acute injury, irradiated marrow cultures, known to have a decreased number of stem cells, grow as well as nonirradiated controls for weeks to months but subsequently display a greatly shortened in vitro life span, presumably due to consumption of their allotted CPD to repopulate the culture during the early recovery phase.[49]

Even if exhaustion of cellular proliferative capacity per se does not occur during normal aging, reduction or loss of a related cellular capacity, such as the ability to respond to specific membrane signals, may contribute to senescence of the organism. Finally, whether or not the in vitro changes associated with increasing tissue donor age can be causally related to aging of the organism, awareness of these cellular phenomena may ultimately facilitate the management of certain clinical disorders in the elderly.

REFERENCES

1. **Carrel, A. and Burrows, M. T.,** Cultivation of tissues in vitro and its technique, *J. Exp. Med.,* 13, 387, 1911.
2. **Carrel, A.,** On the permanent life of tissue outside of the organism, *J. Exp. Med.,* 15, 516, 1912.
3. **Carrel, A.,** Contributing to the study of the mechanism of the growth of connective tissue, *J. Exp. Med.,* 18, 287, 1913.
4. **Carrel, A. and Ebeling, A. H.,** Age and multiplication of fibroblasts, *J. Exp. Med.,* 34, 599, 1921.
5. **Denckla, W. D.,** Role of the pituitary and thyroid glands in the decline of minimal O_2 consumption with age, *J. Clin. Invest.,* 53, 572, 1974.
6. **Parker, R. C.,** *Methods of Tissue Culture,* Harper and Row, New York, 1961.
7. **Hayflick, L. and Moorhead, P. S.,** The serial cultivation of human diploid cell strains, *Exp. Cell Res.,* 25, 585, 1961.
8. **Hayflick, L.,** The limited in vitro lifespan of human diploid cell strains, *Exp. Cell Res.,* 37, 614, 1965.
9. **Hayflick, L.,** The cell biology of aging, *J. Invest. Dermatol.,* 73, 8, 1979.
10. **Hayflick, L.,** The cellular basis for biologic aging, in *Handbook of the Biology of Aging,* Cherkin, A., et al., Eds., Raven Press, New York, 1979, 159.
11. **Daniel, D. W.,** Cell longevity in vivo, in *Handbook of the Biology of Aging,* Cherkin, A., et al., Eds., Raven Press, New York, 1979, 122.
12. **Stanley, J. F., Pye, D., and MacGregor, A.,** Comparison of doubling numbers obtained by cultured animal cells with lifespan of species, *Nature (London),* 255, 158, 1975.
13. **Martin, G. M., Sprague, C. A., and Epstein, C. J.,** Replicative lifespan of cultivated human cells. Effect of donor's age, tissue, and genotype, *Lab. Invest.,* 23, 86, 1970.
14. **Schneider, E. L. and Mitsui, Y.,** The relationship between in vitro cellular aging and in vitro human age, *Proc. Natl. Acad. Sci. USA,* 73, 3584, 1976.
15. **Goldstein, S.,** Lifespan of cultured cells in progeria, *Lancet,* 1, 424, 1969.
16. **Goldstein, S., Littlefield, J. W., and Woeldner, J. S.,** Diabetes mellitus and aging: Diminished plating efficiency of cultured human fibroblasts, *Proc. Natl. Acad. Sci. USA,* 64, 155, 1969.
17. **Goldstein, S. and Moerman, E. J.,** Chronologic and physiologic age effect replicative life-span of fibroblasts from diabetic, prediabetic, and normal donors, *Science,* 199, 781, 1977.
18. **Wojtyk, R. I. and Goldstein, S.,** Fidelity of protein synthesis does not decline during aging of cultured human fibroblasts, *J. Cell. Physiol.,* k03, 299, 1980.
19. **Adelman, R. C.,** Macromolecular metabolism during aging, in *Handbook of the Biology of Aging,* Cherkin, A., et al., Eds., Raven Press, New York, 1979, 63.
20. **Ohno, T.,** Strict relationship between dialyzed serum concentration and cellular lifespan in vitro, *Mech. Aging Dev.,* 11, 179, 1979.
21. **Cristofalo, V. and Rosner, B.,** Modulation of cell proliferation and senescence of WI 38 cells by hydrocortisone, *Fed. Proc. Fed. Am. Soc. Exp. Biol.,* 38, 1851, 1979.
22. **Philips, R. and Cristofalo, V.,** Growth regulation of WI 38 cells in a serum free medium, *Exp. Cell Res.,* 134, 297, 1981.
22a. **Harley, C. B., Goldstein, S., Posner, B. I., and Guyda, H.,** Decreased sensitivity of old and progeric human fibroblasts to a preparation of factors with insulin like activity, *J. Clin. Invest.,* 68, 988, 1981.
22b. **Slaybach, J. R. B., Cheung, L. W. Y., and Geyer, R. P.,** Comparative effect of HPGF on the growth and morphology of human fegal and adult diploid fibroblasts, *Exp. Cell Res.,* 110, 462, 1977.
22c. **Plisko, A. and Gilchrest, B. A.,** Growth factor responsiveness of cultured human fibroblasts declines with age, *J. Gerontol.,* in press.
23. **Rheinwald, J. and Green, H.,** Serial cultivation of strains of human epidermal keratincoytes: the formation of keratinizing colonies from single cells, *Cell,* 6, 331, 1975.
24. **Green, H.,** The keratinocyte as differentiated cell type, *Harvey Lect.,* 74, 101, 1980.

25. **Reinwald, J. and Green, H.,** EGF and the multiplication of cultured human epidermal keratinocytes, *Nature (London),* 265, 421, 1977.

26. **Green, H.,** Cyclic AMP in relation to proliferation of the epidermal cell: new view, *Cell,* 15, 801, 1968.

27. **Gilchrest, B. A.,** Relationship between actinic damage and chronologic aging in keratinocyte cultures in human skin, *J. Invest. Dermatol.,* 72, 219, 1979.

28. **Gilchrest, B. A., Szabo, G., Flynn, E., and Goldwyn, R. M.,** Chronologic and actinically induced aging in human facial skin, *J. Invest. Dermatol.,* 80, 81S, 1983.

29. **Gilchrest, B. A.,** Prior chronic sun exposure decreases the lifespan of human skin fibroblasts in vivo, *J. Gerontol.,* 35, 537, 1980.

30. **Lavker, R. M.,** Structural alterations in exposed and unexposed aged skin, *J. Invest. Dermatol.,* 73, 59, 1979.

30a. **Liu, S. C., Parsons, C. S., and Hanawalt, P. C.,** DNA repair response in human epidermal keratinocytes from donors of different age, *J. Invest. Dermatol.,* 79, 330, 1982.

30b. **Taichman, L. B. and Setlow, R. B.,** Repair of ultraviolet light damage to the DNA of cultured human epidermal keratinocytes and fibroblasts, *J. Invest. Dermatol.,* 73, 217, 1979.

30c. **Hanawalt, P. C., Liu, S. C., and Parsons, C. S.,** DNA repair responses in human skin cells, *J. Invest. Dermatol.,* 77, 86, 1981.

30d. **D'Ambrosio, S. M, Slazinski, L., Whetstone, J. W., and Lowney, E.,** Excision repair of UV-induced pyrimidine dimers in human skin in vivo, *J. Invest. Dermatol.,* 77, 311, 1981.

31. **Gilchrest, B. A.,** In vitro assessment of keratinocyte aging, *J. Invest. Dermatol.,* 81, 184S, 1983.

32. **Merz, G. S. and Ross, J. D.,** Viability of human diploid cells as a function of in vitro age, *J. Cell. Physiol.,* 74, 219, 1969.

33. **Cristofalo, V. J. and Sharf, B. B.,** Cellular senescence and DNA synthesis (thymidine incorporation as a measure of population age in human diploid cells), *Exp. Cell Res.,* 76, 419, 1973.

34. **Smith, J. R., Pereira-Smith, O., and Good, P. I.,** Colony size distribution as a measure of age in cultured human cells. A brief note, *Mech. Aging Dev.,* 6, 283, 1977.

35. **Bell, E., Marek, L. F., Levinstone, D. S., Merrill, C., Sher, S., Young, I. T., and Eden, M.,** Loss of division potential in vitro: Aging or differentiation?, *Science,* 202, 1158, 1978.

36. **Green, H., Kehinde, O., and Thomas, J.,** Formation of abundant viable epithelium by cultured human epidermal cells and its possible use for grafting, *Proc. Natl. Acad. Sci. USA,* 76, 5665, 1979.

37. **Gilchrest, B. A., Calhoun, J. K., and Maciag, T.,** Attachment and growth of human keratincoytes in a serum free environment, *J. Cell. Physiol.,* 112, 197, 1982.

38. **Eisinger, M., and Marko, O.,** Selective proliferation of normal human melanocytes in vitro in the presence of phorol ester and cholera toxin, *Proc. Natl. Acad. Sci. USA,* 79, 2018, 1982.

39. **Wilkins, L. M., Gilchrest, B. A., Maciag, T., Szabo, G., and Connell, L.,** Growth of enriched human melanocyte cultures, in *Growth of Cells in Hormonally Defined Media,* Sato, G. H., et al., Eds., *Cold Spring Harbor Conferences on Cell Proliferation,* Vol. 9, 1982, 929.

40. **Folkman, J., Haudenschild, C. C., and Zetter, B. R.,** Long term culture of capillary endothelial cells, *Proc. Natl. Acad. Sci. USA,* 76, 5217, 1979.

41. **Sherer, G. K., Fitzharris, T. P., Faulk, W. P., and LeRoy, E. C.,** Cultivation of microvasculature endothelial cells from human preputial skin, *In Vitro,* 16, 675, 1980.

42. **Maciag, T., Hoover, G., Stemerman, M. B., and Weinstein, R.,** Human endothelial cell growth control in vitro, *J. Cell Biol.,* 91, 420, 1981.

43. **Davidson, P. M., Bensch, K., and Karasek, M. A.,** Isolation and growth of endothelial cells from the microvessels of the newborn human foreskin in cell culture, *J. Invest. Dermatol.,* 75, 316, 1980.

44. **Maciag, T., Weinstein, R., Stemerman, M., and Gilchrest, B. A.,** Selective growth of human endothelial cells from both papillary and reticular dermis, *J. Invest. Dermatol.,* 74, 256, 1980.

45. **Duthu, G. S. and Smith, J. R.,** In vitro proliferation and lifespan of bovine aorta endothelial cells: Effects of culture conditions and fibroblast growth factor, *J. Cell. Physiol.,* 103, 385, 1980.

46. **Mueller, S. N., Rosen, E. M., and Levine, E. M.,** Cellular senescence in a cloned strain of bovine fetal aortic endothelial cells, *Science,* 207, 889, 1980.

47. **Fitzpatrick, T. B., Szabo, G., and Mitchell, R.,** Age changes in the human melanocyte system, in *Advances in the Biology of the Skin,* Montagna, W., et al., Eds., Pergamon Press, Oxford, 1964, 35.

Chapter 8

DERMATOHELIOSIS (SUN-INDUCED AGING)

I. INTRODUCTION

Dermatoheliosis is a term coined* to describe the array of clinical and histological findings which characterize chronically sun-exposed skin in middle-aged and elderly adults. Initially due to ignorance of its true pathophysiology and more recently due to lack of an appropriate word, dermatoheliosis has been widely mislabeled in both the lay and medical literature as "aging", "premature aging", or "accelerated aging". It is indeed this confusion between the process of chronic sun damage and intrinsic aging, rather than any biologic relationship, that motivates the inclusion of dermatoheliosis in a treatise on cutaneous aging.

II. HISTORICAL PERSPECTIVE

Less than 20 years ago, the alteration of dermal elastin fibers observed both clinically and microscopically in habitually sun-exposed skin commonly was known as "senile elastosis",[1] and a paper documenting the more direct association with sun exposure than with advanced age warranted publication in a major medical journal.[2] Even in current dermatology texts, aging is often relegated to sections dealing primarily with the effects of light on the skin.[3]

A second etiologic confusion of historical interest is evident in the original description of cutis rhomboidalis nuchae. The presence of this striking cutaneous abnormality on the posterior neck of multiple family members led Nikolsky to postulate that the lesion itself was hereditary,[4] not the patients' underlying fair complexion and outdoor occupations (the former genetically determined and the latter societally determined).

III. CLINICAL FEATURES

Clinical features of actinically damaged skin are listed in Table 1. The relative severity of these changes varies considerably among individuals, undoubtedly reflecting inherent differences in vulnerability and repair capacity for the solar insult. All occur predominantly in fair-skinned Caucasians with a history of ample past sun-exposure and usually involve the face, neck, or extensor surface of the upper extremities most severely.[5-7] The apparent influence of sex on the prevalence of certain of these conditions undoubtedly reflects in part different hair styles, patterns of dress and nature of sun exposure (occupational vs. recreational) between men and women over the past several generations; other sex differences such as epidermal thickness[8] and sebaceous gland activity[9] may also influence their development. The characteristic distribution of lesions in each condition is a complex function of relative insolation for different body sites, anatomic distribution of the participating cutaneous structures (e.g., melanocytes and sebaceous glands), and other poorly understood factors. Genetic determinants beyond those for melanin synthetic capacity are undoubtedly operative.

By definition, these changes are due to repeated sun exposure, but the more detailed pathophysiology is in all cases speculative. Incompletely repairable cumulative damage to

---

* Dr. Thomas B. Fitzpatrick deserves credit for repeated efforts to introduce this useful term into dermatologic parlance.

Table 1
FEATURES OF ACTINICALLY DAMAGED SKIN

Clinical abnormalities	Histologic abnormality	Presumed pathophysiology
Dryness (roughness)	Minimal stratum corneum irregularity	Altered keratinocyte maturation
Actinic keratoses	Nuclear atypia; loss of orderly, progressive keratinocyte maturation; irregular epidermal hyper- and/or hypoplasia; occasional dermal inflammation	Premalignant disorder
Irregular pigmentation		
Freckling	Reduced number of hypertrophied, strongly dopa-positive melanocytes	Reactive hyperplasia and later loss of functional melanocytes
Lentigenes	Elongation of epidermal rete ridges; increase in number and melanization of melanocytes	
Guttate hypomelanosis	Absence of melanocytes	

Dermis

Wrinkling		
Fine surface lines	None detected	Alterations in dermal matrix and fibrous proteins
Deep furrows		
Stellate pseudo-scars	Absence of epidermal pigmentation, altered dermal collagen	Loss of functional melanocytes, reactive collagen deposition by fibroblasts
Elastosis (fine nodularity and/or coarseness)	Nodular aggregations of fibrous to amorphorous material in the papillary dermis	Overproduction of abnormal elastin fibers
Inelasticity	Elastotic dermis	Altered elastin fibers
Telaniectasia	Ectatic vessels often with atrophic walls	Loss of connective tissue support
Venous lakes	Ectatic vessels often with atrophic walls	Loss of connective tissue support
Purpura (easy bruising)	Extravasated erythrocytes	Loss of connective tissue support for dermal vessel walls

Appendages

Comedones (Maladie de Favre et Racouchot)	Ectatic superficial portion of the pilosebaceous follicle	Loss of connective tissue support
Sebaceous hyperplasia	Concentric hyperplasia of sebaceous glands	Increased mitotic and functional responsiveness of glandular tissue

the skin's cellular constituents with subsequent inability to perform their differentiated functions is the logical primary event.

In the epidermis, injury to basal keratinocytes is presumed to result in an altered morphology and a defective maturation program for the terminally differentiated daughter cells, with the clinical and histologic consequences of an irregular, "scaly" stratum corneum and multiple actinic keratoses (Figure 1 and Plate 8).* The mild to moderate inflammation which accompanies many actinic keratoses[10] may indicate a low-grade immunologic reaction to altered keratinocyte surface antigens or simply a response to on-going cellular injury. The striking epidermal atrophy sometimes seen in chronically sun-exposed skin may reflect depletion of cells in the germinative compartment.[11]

---

*   Plate 8 appears after page 100.

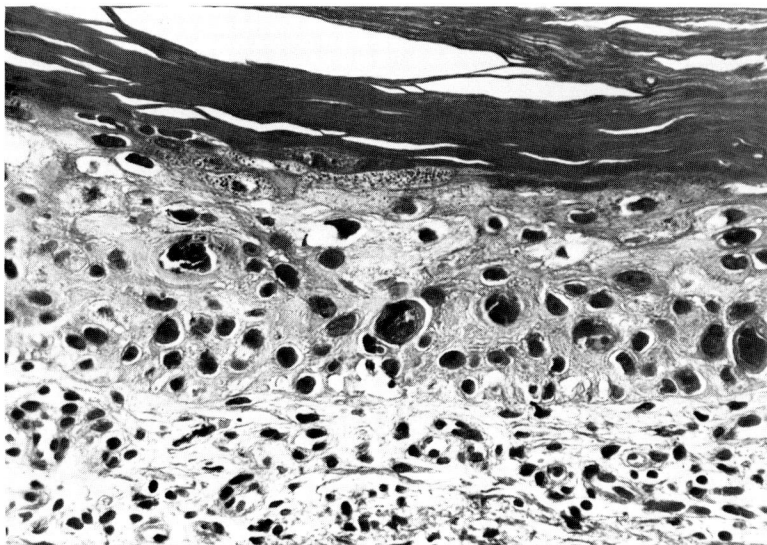

FIGURE 1. Actinic keratoses. Histologic features of an actinic keratosis. Note thick stratum corneum, atrophic epidermis, cellular atypia, and disorderly arrangement of keratinocytes with variable staining in routine preparation. Lesions may also be hyperplastic or even occasionally bullous. (Section kindly selected and photographed by Theodore Kwan, M. D. and Roxanne Lucero, M.D.)

The virtually universal irregularity of epidermal pigmentation which characterizes sun-damaged Caucasian skin is due in part to reactive hyperplasia and subsequent depletion of the injured melanocytes and perhaps in part to impaired pigment transfer to keratinocytes. This process is most clearly reflected in freckles (ephilides) which contain a decreased number of large, highly dendritic, strongly dopa-positive melanocytes.[11] The guttate hypomelanosis commonly seen on the lower legs may represent a further evolution in which loss of functional melanocytes dominates the clinical picture. In contrast, "senile" or "solar" lentigenes are characterized by an increased number and increased pigment production of epidermal melanocytes[12] (Figure 2 and Plate 9).* The associated elongation of epidermal rete ridges suggests keratinocytic and/or fibroblastic participation in this lesion, which may conceivably account for the prominent melanocyte activity. The much less common lentigo maligna differs in being a well-established precursor to invasive melanoma with histologically atypical actively proliferating melanocytes[13,14] (Figure 3 and Plate 10),* although the inciting event is also actinically induced cellular injury.

In the dermis, fibroblast injury appears to underlie most or all of the clinical changes of dermatoheliosis. Both fine "surface lines" and deep furrows in the sites of frequent skin flexure are widely presumed to result from changes in elastin and/or collagen fibers and possibly from changes in the dermal ground substance, although precise histologic concomitants of wrinkling have never been identified. A classic clinical presentation is cutis rhomboidalis nuchae (Plate 11).*

Elastosis, the pebbly or "goose flesh" quality often most prominent on the lateral neck and upper chest, is due to nodular aggregations of altered elastin fibers in the dermis[2,16] (Figure 4). The process is progressively more prevalent with each decade in both lightly and darkly pigmented populations, and among fair-skinned Caucasians severe histologic

* Plates 9, 10, and 11 appear after page 100.

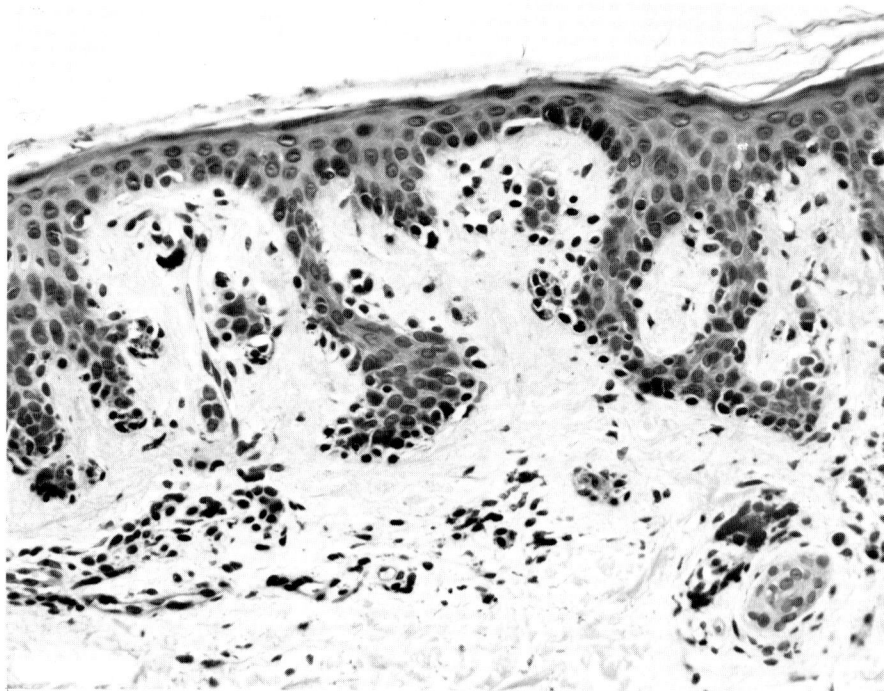

FIGURE 2.   Solar lentigo. Histologic features of a lentigo. Note epidermal hyperpigmentation and deeply convoluted dermo-epidermal junction with thin club-shaped rete. The intervening epidermis is atrophic. (Section kindly selected and photographed by Theodore Kwan, M.D. and Roxanne Lucero, M.D.)

damage is univerally present by the sixth decade[16a] (Figure 5). In formalin-fixed hematoxylin and eosin-stained sections under the light microscope, fibrous to amorphous material with altered tinctorial properties occupies predominantly the papillary dermis below a narrow, apparently spared Grenz zone.[16-18] Verhoeff-stained sections demonstrate a proliferation of elastin fibers.[18] In severely sun-damaged skin, an increased number of thickened, tangled elastin fibers occupy both the papillary and reticular dermis.[18] At much higher magnifications, this material can be resolved into a variable number of abnormal fibrils and extensive granular amorphous material which appears histochemically to represent elastin rather than collagen.[19,20] In one study, a 5 to 20-fold increase in elastic fiber diameter with slight changes in fibrillar ultrastructure was detected in mildly sun-damaged skin, compared to age-matched sun-protected skin.[18] Elastin fibers in skin severely involved by clinical criteria were disrupted and "moth-eaten" with loss of their normal architecture, there was no morphologic evidence of collagen participation in the elastosis.[18] Elastic fiber alterations in aged sun-protected skin were qualitatively different and could be mimicked by elastase or chymotrypsin digestion of young skin, while solar elastosis could not[18] (see also Chapter 3). In a separate study, the Grenz zone routinely observed above elastotic areas in the dermis contained densely packed collagen fibrils in a co-linear arrangement parallel to the skin surface and therefore probably a "microscar" rather than an area of sparing.[17] Inelasticity or lack of elastic recoil in sun-damaged skin is a biophysical rather than histologic change, but is strongly associated with the above morphologic abnormalities of dermal elastin fibers.

   The overall impression from available studies is one of progressive injury to dermal fibroblasts in habitually sun-exposed skin, eventually resulting in dysfunctional, quantitative,

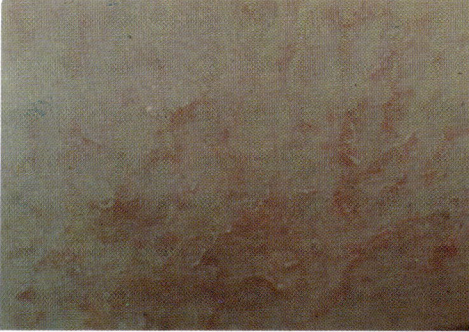

PLATE 1. Erythema craquele. Superficial erythematous fissures on leg partially outline "squamous islands" within the stratum corneum. (Photograph courtesy of Neil A. Fenske, M.D.)

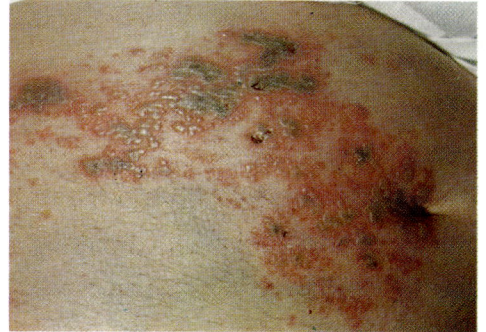

PLATE 2. Herpes zoster. Clear grouped vesicles, pustules, and hemorrhagic vesicles superimposed on erythematous plaques involve the left T 10 dermatome. Lesions begin in the midline posteriorly and end abruptly at the umbilicus anteriorly. There is usually considerable pain and hyperesthesia of the affected skin during the first days of the illness, and a Tzank smear should be floridly positive.

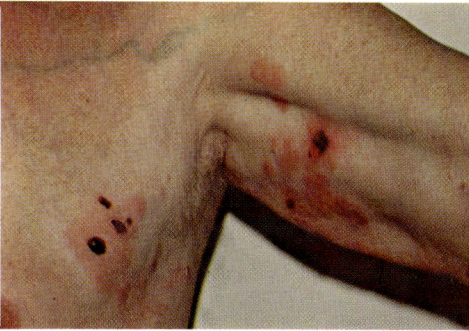

A

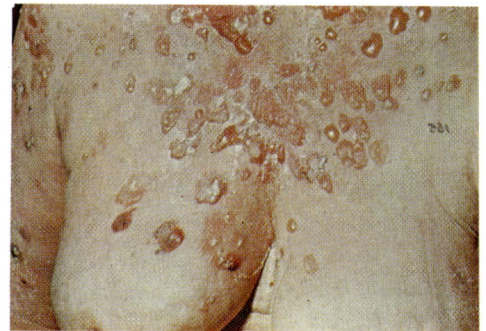

B

PLATE 3. Bullous pemphigoid (BP). (A) Hemorrhagic bullae and crusted erosions arising on erythematous plaques involve the chest and arm. (Photograph courtesy of Neil A. Fenske, M.D.) (B) Multiple tense and flaccid bullae, some hemorrhagic, arising from normal-appearing skin are also characteristic of BP. (Photograph courtesy of Kenneth A. Arndt, M.D.)

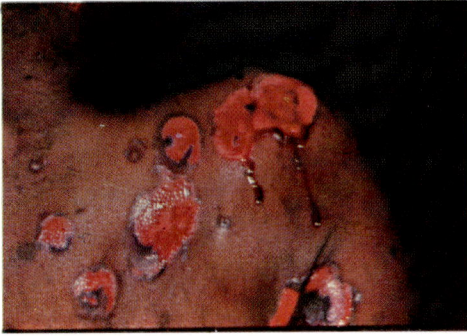

PLATE 4. Pemphigus vulgaris (PV). Large erosions involve the scapular area. Intact bullae are not present. Normal-appearing skin adjacent to lesions may slough with minor trauma. In the absence of treatment, re-epitheliazation is rare. (Photograph courtesy of Neil A. Fenske, M.D.)

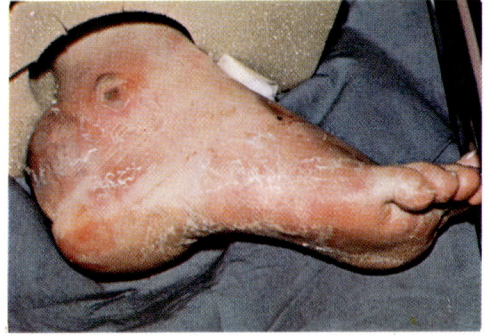

PLATE 5. Pressure bullae. Large tense blisters are apparent over the heel and lateral malleolus as a result of prolonged direct weight-bearing on these sites. (Photograph courtesy of Neil A. Fenske, M.D.)

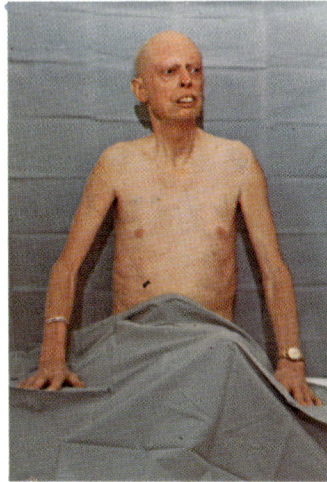

A

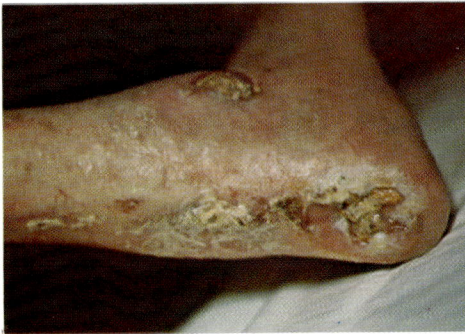

B

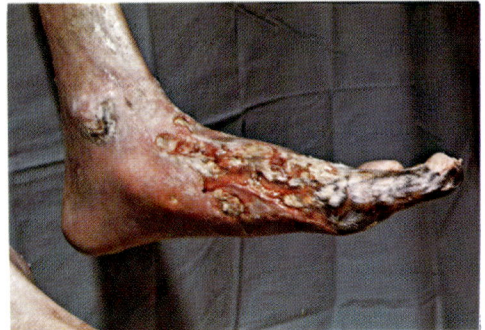

C

PLATE 6. Werner Syndrome. (A) Fifty-two-year-old man with balding, generalized sclerosis, "taut" facies, and atrophic musculature. (B) Patient's right heel, showing cutaneous atrophy and sclerosis, complicated by deep non-heeling ulcerations over the os calcis and lateral maleolus. (C) Patient's left foot, showing sclerosis, deep ulceration, and gangrene of the entire hallux. Mid-thigh amputation was eventually required. (Photographs kindly supplied by J. A. Zalla, M.D. and reprinted with permission from Zalla, J. A., Cutis, 25, 275, 1980.)

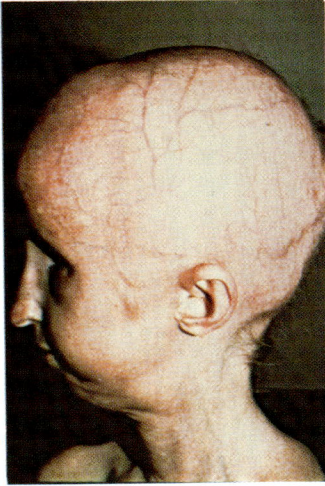
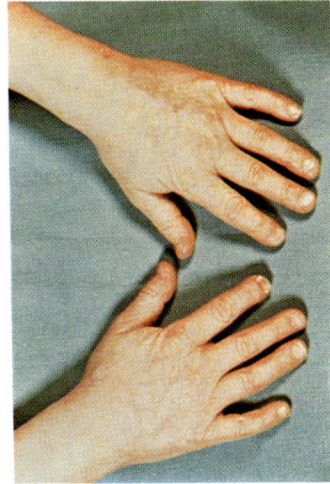

A   B

PLATE 7. Progeria. (A) Profile of a 13-year-old boy demonstrating craniofacial disproportion, micrograthia, almost total alopecia, and prominent venous pattern on the scalp. (B) Patient's hands, demonstrating lax finely wrinkled skin. (Photographs kindly supplied by G. M. Martin, M.D. and reproduced with permission from Martin, G. M., Sprague, C. A., and Epstein, C. J., Lab. Invest., 23, 86, 1970.)

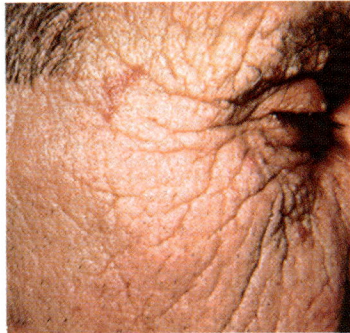

PLATE 8. Actinic keratoses. Irregular thin red plaque on the right temple of a man with severe elastosis and other evidence of sun damage. The area is rough to palpation but otherwise asymptomatic. (Photograph courtesy of Steven Shama, M.D.)

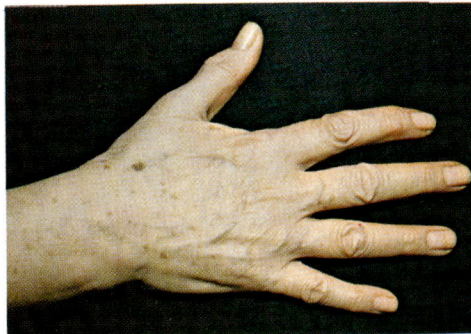

PLATE 9. Solar lentigo. Dark brown macule on the dorsum of the hand, also called an "age spot." Numerous light tan lentigenes are also present.

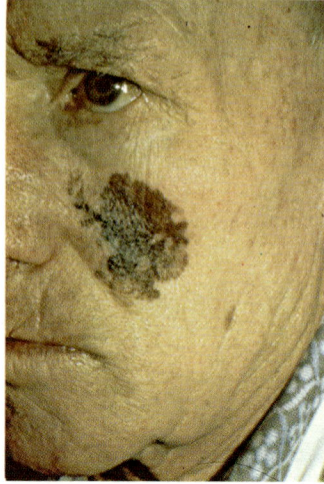

PLATE 10.   Lentigo maligna. Large irregularly shaped
brown to black macule involving the left cheek. The
lesion is slowly enlarging and asymptomatic. Surrounding skin is moderately sun damaged.

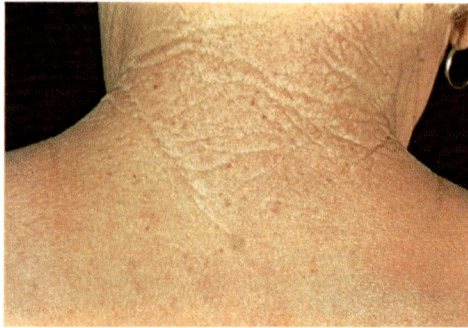

PLATE 11. Cutis rhomboidalis nuchae. Deep criss-
crossing furrows and an overall ''pebbly'' quality of the
skin are apparent on the posterior neck.

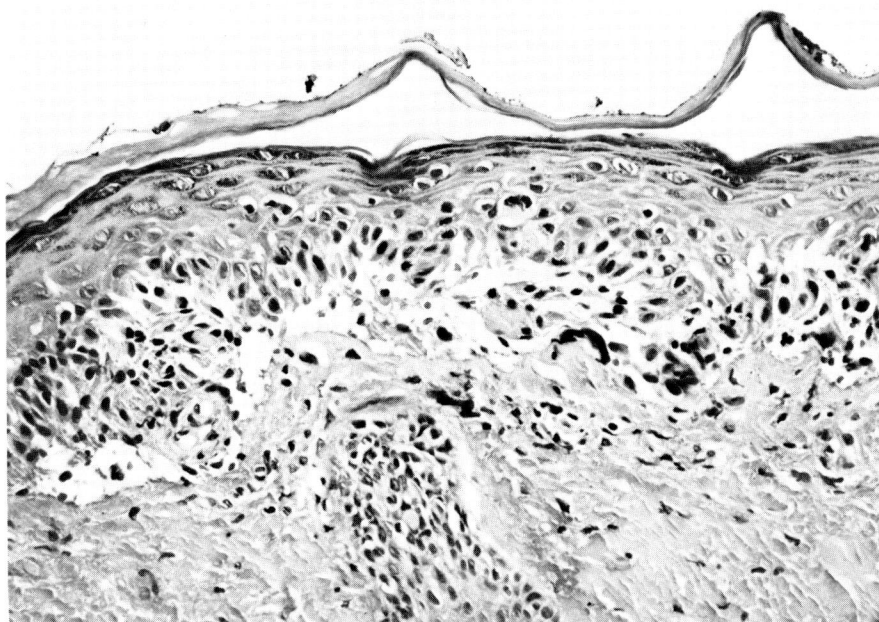

FIGURE 3. Lentigo maligna. Histologic features of lentigo maligna. Numerous large atypical melanocytes are located singly and in nests along the basal layer of the epidermis, separated from the dermis by an artifactual cleft. Invasion into the dermis is absent. (Section kindly selected and photographed by Theodore Kwan, M.D. and Roxanne Lucero, M.D.)

and qualitative alterations of collagen and elastin. The striking vertical gradient of change, most severe in the papillary dermis and less severe in the deeper reticular dermis, is consistent with the attenuation of solar energy as it passes through skin (vide infra).

Less is known about the pathogenesis of the vascular lesions in dermatoheliosis. All occur in elastotic dermis, and altered perivenular connective tissue may well provide less support, resulting in ectatic superficial vessels, but direct injury to endothelial cells and other components of the vessel wall cannot be excluded. A careful electron-microscopic study of actinically damaged skin *not* selected for clinically apparent vascular changes revealed marked thickening of postcapillary venular walls due to concentric deposition of basement membrane-like material admixed with collagen (reticulin) fibers,[21] identical to that noted in the skin of porphyric patients.[22] Histological evidence suggested synthesis of the material by perivenular veil cells.[21] Biopsies from sun-protected skin of the four oldest subjects studied 80 to 93 years, revealed 50 to 80% thinning of postcapillary venular walls with partial to complete loss of surrounding veil cells, compared to sun-protected skin of young adults.[21] Biopsies from sun-damaged skin of these individuals were unfortunately unavailable, however. Actinically induced facial telangiectasia, venous lakes, and "senile" purpura of the extensor forearms have apparently not been studied in comparable detail.

Of the appendageal lesions associated with dermatoheliosis, open and closed comedones involving the face (Maladie de Favre et Racouchot[23] or nodular cutaneous elastoidosis with cysts and comedones[24]) has the least disputable relationship to actinic damage. The lesions occur most frequently along the infraorbital ridge and on the temples of fair-skinned Caucasian males with ample past sun exposure. Histologically, the lesions are greatly dilated

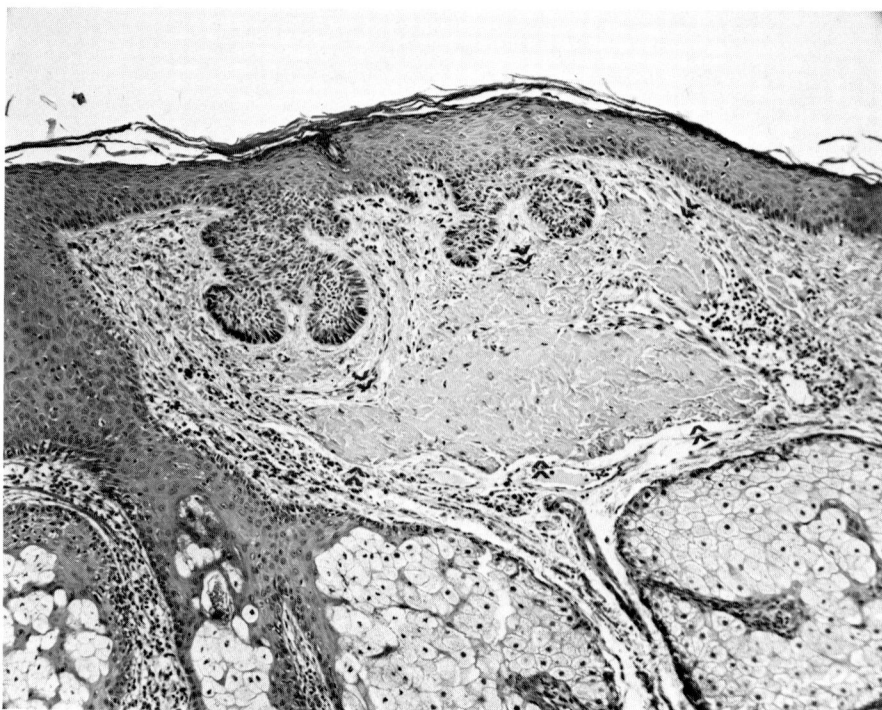

FIGURE 4.   Solar elastosis. An aggregate of altered elastin fibers (area within the double ''v'' marks) is present in the upper dermis below an area of apparent sparing. In hemotoxylin and eosin-stained sections, the altered material is blue, in contrast to the normal pink dermis. Foci of basal cell carcinoma overlie the elastosis. Large sebaceous gland is characteristic of facial skin. (Section kindly selected and photographed by Theodore Kwan, M.D. and Roxanne Lucero, M.D.)

pilosebaceous follicles with atrophic sebaceous glands set in an elastotic dermis.[24] The clinical and histologic features are consistent with gradual ectasia of the follicles secondary to loss of connective tissue support. Sebaceous hyperplasia, characterized clinically by soft yellowish papules with central umbilication, also seems more common among fair-skinned than among dark-skinned individuals, and occurs almost exclusively on the face, usually the forehead.[25] Histologically, each papule consists of one or a few hyperplastic multilobulated glands concentrically arranged about an enlarged duct. In contrast to the other dermal components of dermatoheliosis, the lesions appear to result from true hyperplasia rather than ectasia of existing structures.

Quantitative data regarding the effects of aging and habitual sun exposure are available for two types of epidermal cells, melanocytes and Langerhans cells (LC). An approximately 20% increase in dopa-positive melanocytes/mm^2 was measured in biopsies of the lateral (sun-exposed) aspect of the arm in eight adult Caucasian volunteers, aged 28 to 80 years, who had no recent sun exposure[26] (Figure 6). Differences in melanocyte size and dendricity between the two sites were variable and much less striking than differences in cell density. This *increase* in melanocyte density attributable to habitual sun exposure contrasts with the *decrease* observed as a function of advancing donor age in both biopsy sites (Figure 7).

As noted in Chapter 3, an age-associated reduction in the density of epidermal LC was noted in a histologic study comparing sun-protected buttock skin of four young (22 to 26 year old) and seven old (62 to 86 year old) subjects.[27] Another study, designed to examine

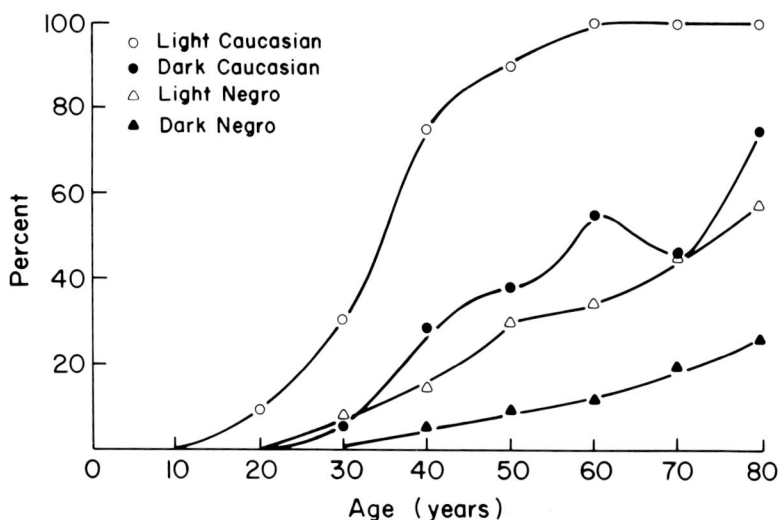

FIGURE 5. Prevalence of elastosis by age. Punch biopsies of skin from the malar eminence were stained with the elastic tissue stain orcein and graded on a 0 to 4 scale for severity of elastosis. The percent in each 10-year age cohort with grade 3 or 4 (severe) elastosis is plotted for four groups of varying skin color. (The values for volunteers aged 21 to 30 years are plotted on the ordinate at 30 years, and so forth. Each point represents a cohort of 10 to 58 (most 20 to 40) volunteers, all residents of Philadelphia). Severe elastosis is universally present in fair-skinned Caucasians by the sixth decade and affects nearly 30% of dark-skinned Blacks by age 80 years. In sunnier climates, age-specific prevalence figures might be higher. (Modified and reproduced with permission from Kligman, A. M., *Sunlight and Man*, Pathak, M. A., et al., Eds., University of Tokyo Press, Tokyo, 1974, 157.)

the effect of habitual sun exposure on epidermal LC, revealed a more than 50% average reduction in LC number for pre-auricular (sun-exposed) vs. post-auricular (sun-protected) surgical specimens obtained from seven middle-aged women undergoing rhydidectomies (face lifts).[28] Similar results have been reported for paired sun-exposed and nonexposed nuchal sites in men with severely sun-damaged skin.[29] Of interest, the changes in both melanocyte and LC density attributable to chronic sun exposure may be viewed as a perpetuation of the acute changes induced by solar or other UV irradiation.

IV. RESPONSIBLE PORTION OF THE SOLAR SPECTRUM

Although ambient sun exposure is unquestionably (and by definition) responsible for dermatoheliosis, the relative contribution of various spectral bands is unknown. The necessary experiments have never been performed because of the extremely long time required for manifestation of the disorder in man (usually more than 30 years), and because, due to species differences in cutaneous structure, there is no truly appropriate animal model. Studies utilizing mice[30,31] and rats[32] have demonstrated that an elastosis-like condition can be produced by prolonged irradiation with a predominantly UVB source (vide infra), but do not examine the relative efficacy of longer wavelengths. Epidemiologic data for man have not been examined in this regard because regional differences in the composition of sunlight (i.e., the relative proportions of different spectral bands) are dwarfed by differences in overall intensity and by racial and occupational differences among prospective study populations.

Solar irradiation reaching the surface of the earth has been classified into convenient bands, largely according to the known effects of the radiation on human tissue:[33] ultraviolet

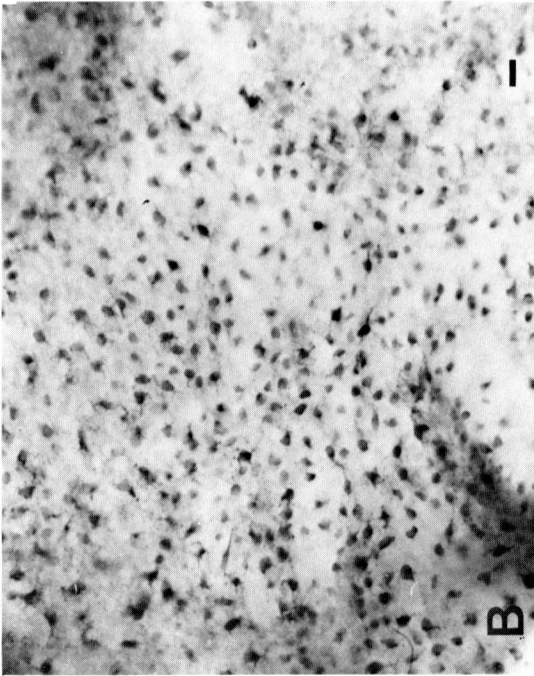

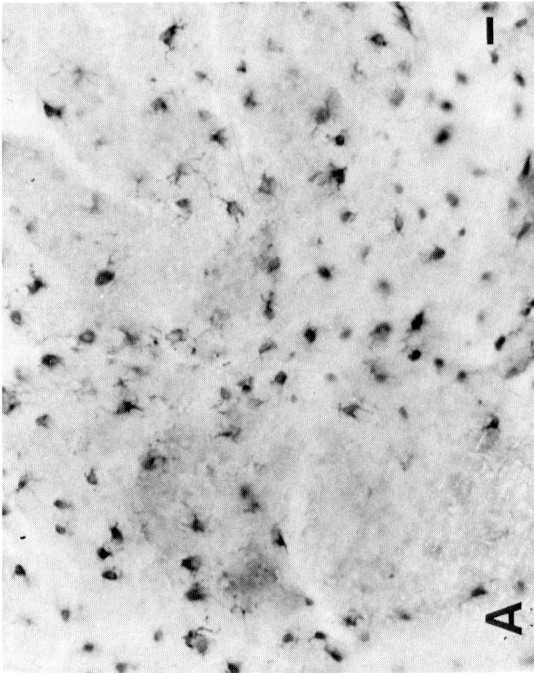

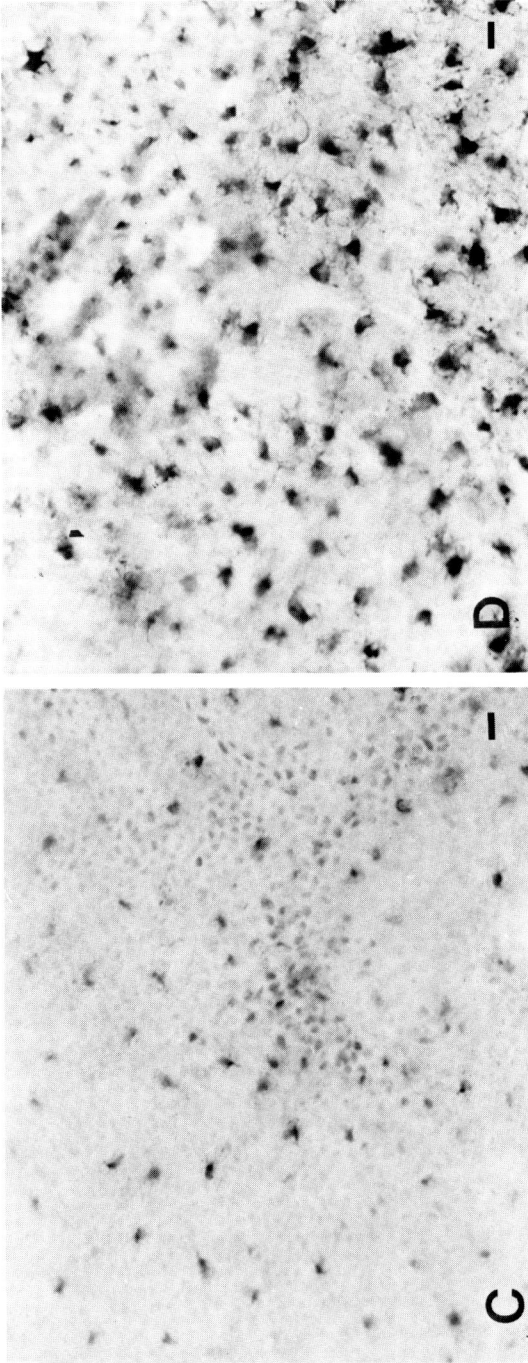

C

D

FIGURE 6. Effect of habitual sun exposure on epidermal melanocytes. Trypsin-split epidermal fragments were incubated in dopa (L-3,4-dihydroxyphenyl-alanine) to stain melanocytes. Biopsies from the medial (A) and lateral (B) aspects of the upper arm of a 61-year-old donor. Note increased number and greater dopa-positivity of melanocytes in (B). Biopsies from the medial (C) and lateral (D) aspects of the upper arm of a 71-year-old donor. Note increased number, larger size, and greater dendricity of melanocytes in (D). Neither subject's arm had been exposed to the sun for at least 6 months; both were fair-skinned Caucasians with moderately severe dermatoheliosis. Scale bars 10 μm. (Reproduced with permission from Gilchrest, B. A., et al., *J. Invest. Dermatol.*, 73, 141, 1979.)

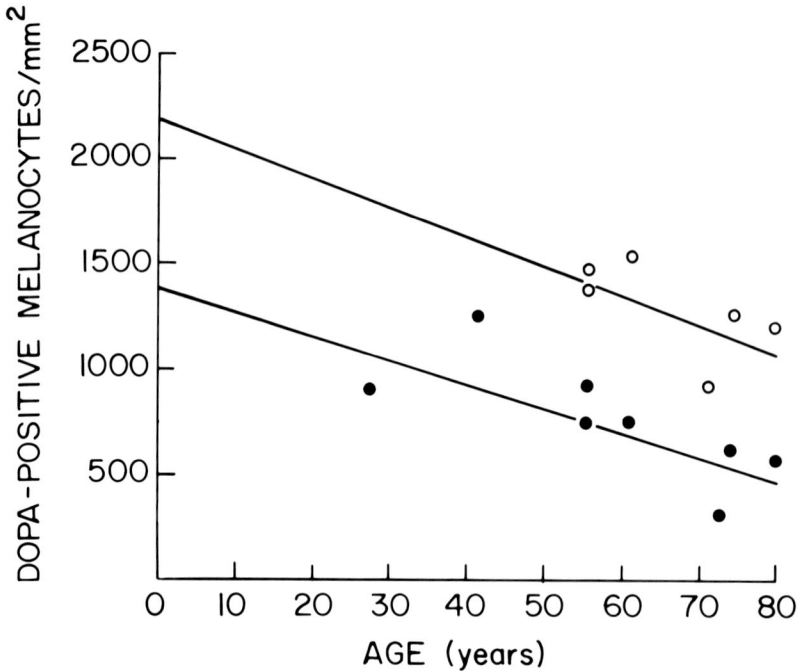

FIGURE 7.   Relationship between age and melanocyte density in habitually sun-exposed skin of the lateral arm (open circles) and nonexposed skin of the medial arm (closed circles) in well-screened fair-skinned adult volunteers without recent sun exposure. Melanocyte counts are the average for 10 independent fields of each split-dopa preparation, viewed at 25× magnification. The density of dopa-positive cells declines approximately 6 to 8% per decade in both sites, but is consistently higher in habitually (previously) sun-exposed skin. (Reproduced with permission from Gilchrest, B. A., et al., *J. Invest. Dermatol.*, 73, 141, 1979.)

(UV) light, visible light, infrared (heat) energy, and radiowaves (Figure 8). The UV spectrum is further subdivided into UV-C (200 to 290 nm), those wavelengths absorbed by ozone; UVB (290 to 320 nm), those wavelengths blocked by glass, primarily responsible for the sunburn reaction and for photocarcinogenesis;[36] and UV-A (290 to 400 nm), those wavelengths largely transmitted through glass and responsible for most photosensitization reactions in the human skin.[33]

Within the 290 to 1000 nm range, particles of light or "photons" with shorter wavelength and higher frequency are more "energetic."[33] This relationship is given mathematically by the formulae $E = hv$ and $\lambda = 1/v$, where E = energy, v = frequency, λ = wavelength, and h is a constant (Planck's constant). More energetic photons with shorter wavelengths are more capable of interacting photochemically with biologic molecules than are those with longer wavelengths, and hence are responsible for most of the recognized effects of UV radiation on DNA, collagen, and other specific cutaneous targets. Average depth of penetration of light into human skin is also determined in large part by its electromagnetic properties, with longer wavelengths penetrating more deeply[33] (Figure 9).

These reciprocal characteristics of light, energy per photon and depth of penetration into skin, form the crux of the debate regarding dermatoheliosis. In the absence of more data, it is impossible to determine whether the changes are caused by the relatively few high energy UV-B photons reaching the basal layer of the epidermis and deeper dermal structures, the more numerous UV-A photons, or indeed the even more numerous visible and infrared photons. (To make even these crude calculations, it is necessary to consider both the relative number of photons in each spectral band of sunlight (Figure 9) and the percent of incident

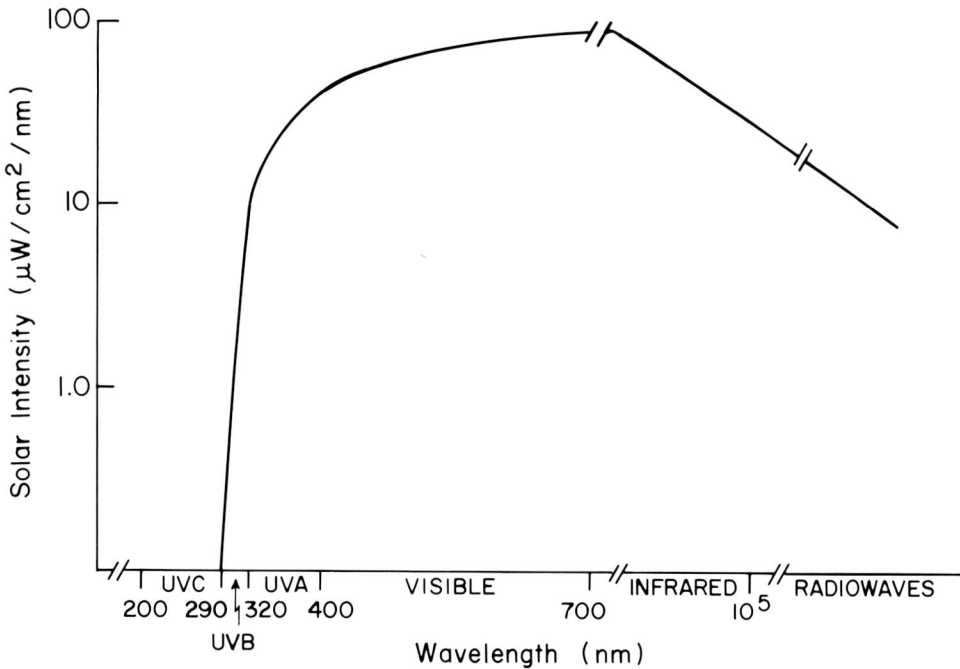

FIGURE 8.   Solar irradiance. The electromagnetic energy incident on the surface of the earth is shown schematically as a function of wavelength and the arbitrarily defined spectral bands. The exact shape of the curve depends upon latitude, altitude, season, and weather conditions, although the energy ratios for UVB:UVA:total remain approximately 0.5:5:100. Hence, only a small fraction of man's sun exposure is to the UV portion of the spectrum.

photons reaching a given depth in the skin (Figure 10)). Furthermore, this approach implicitly assumes that dermatoheliosis has approximately the same action spectrum as sunburn,[36] that is, that higher energy photons are disproportionately more efficient than lower energy longer wavelength photons in producing these lesions.[37] At present no data support this assumption. Indeed, anecdotal reports suggest that repeated infrared irradiation in doses producing no other delayed sequelae may be capable of severely altering the dermal matrix in a manner clinically and histologically reminiscent of dermatoheliosis.[72]

In summary, although UV-B is widely assumed to be responsible for the long-term adverse cutaneous effects of solar radiation, available data by no means exclude a major role for UV-A or even longer wavelengths.

V. LABORATORY INVESTIGATIONS

Early biochemical studies of chronically sun-exposed human skin revealed increased hexosamine and decreased hydroxyproline compared to sun-protected skin,[38] changes contrary to those previously reported to accompany aging (maturation) in sun-protected skin.[39] The pattern observed was believed consistent with the increase in elastin content of actinically damaged skin, determined biochemically to be approximately fourfold by one small study,[40] since this protein has far less hydroxyproline than collagen,[41] the major protein by weight. Compared to relatively sun-protected abdominal skin of adult controls aged 24 to 74 years, clinically sun-damaged forearm skin, per 100 mg dry weight, had more than 4 times the nonfibrous protein, twice the soluble collagen, and approximately half the insoluble collagen and total collagen.[42] These findings suggested increased degradation and/or increased turnover of new collagen in habitually exposed skin. The amino acid composition of material

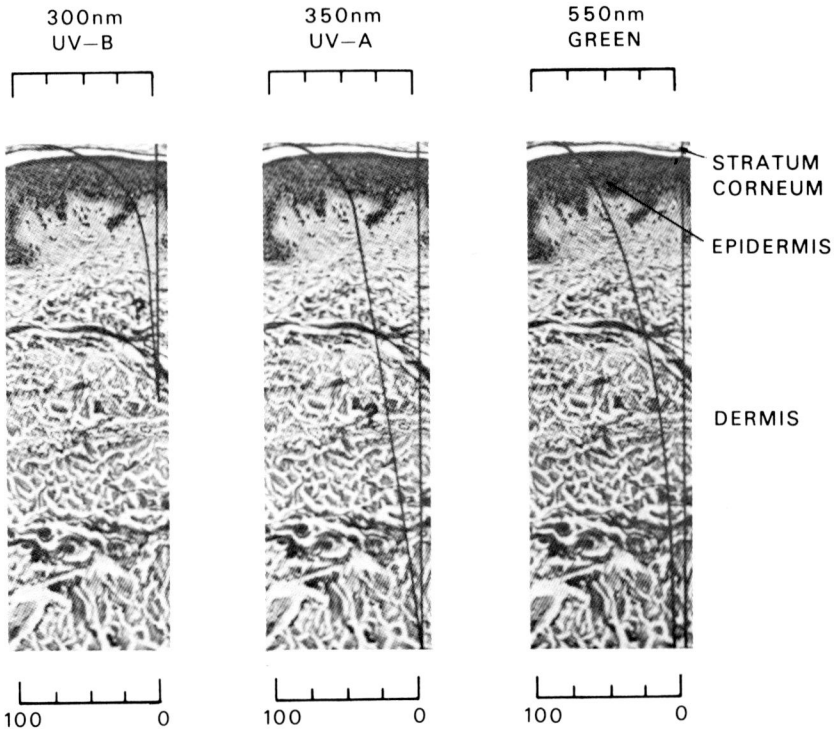

FIGURE 9

determined by extraction to be elastin did not differ between sun-protected and sun-exposed adult skin,[42] arguing against the possibility that "elastosis" represented altered collagen rather than elastin.

Elastosis was produced experimentally in shaved albino mice by 3 months of UV irradiation, sufficiently intense to kill 50% of the animals and to produce tumors in a few, and to a lesser degree by twice weekly application of the irritant promotor croton oil.[30] The increased elastin apparent histologically could not be detected biochemically, but the elastotic dermis did manifest a marked decrease in insoluble collagen,[30] a pattern also present in sun-damaged human skin.[42] A second investigation utilizing shaved albino rats produced elastosis by histologic and histochemical criteria with 6 months of repeated UV irradiation sufficient to cause ulceration, alopecia, and scarring.[32] Elastic tissue was virtually absent immediately after the irradiation period, a finding attributed to destruction of connective tissue by the prolonged UV-induced inflammation, but there was progressive accumulation of normal to thickened elastin fibers during the subsequent 19 weeks of the study. Telangiectasia (dilation and tortuosity of small dermal vessels) and increased acid mucopolysaccharide in ground substance were also noted in the irradiated rat skin.[32]

These early findings have been confirmed and expanded by recent histologic and histochemical experiments.[31,43,44] In the most comprehensive study, hairless mice were exposed three times weekly for 30 weeks to a dose of UVB sufficient to produce tumors in all the animals.[31] Elastic tissue stains of irradiated skin revealed a greatly increased number of thickened, tangled fibers throughout the dermis. These were associated with an increased number of enlarged mast cells and histologically activated fibroblasts, a marked increase in acid mycopolysaccharides and a compensatory loss of collagen. Within weeks after the

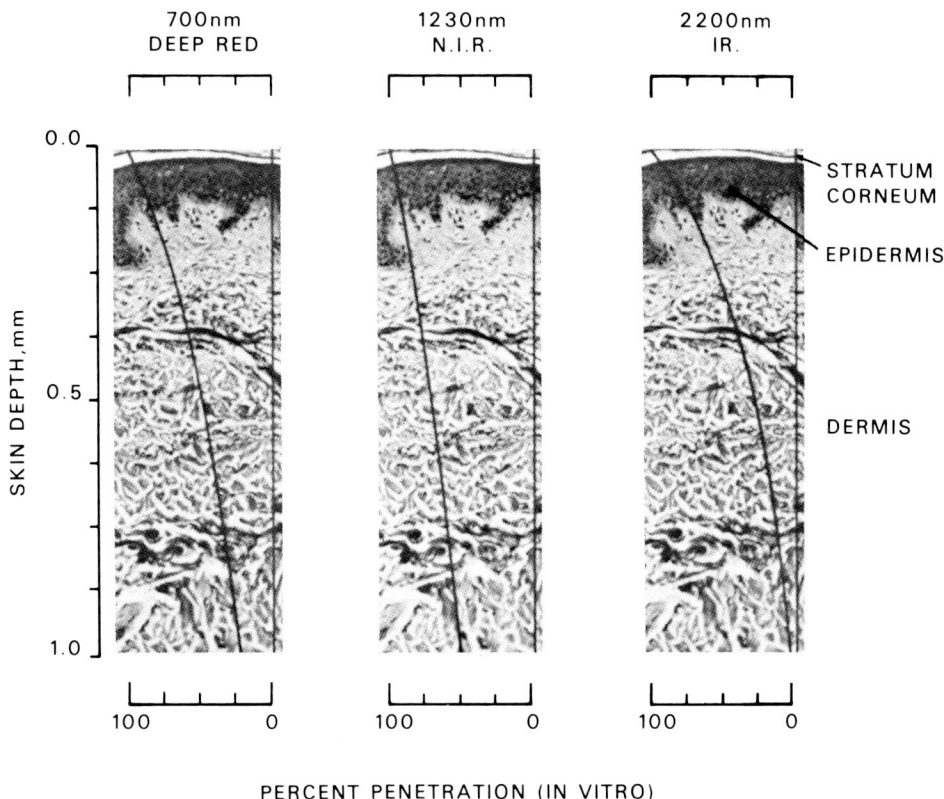

FIGURE 9. Diagrammatic summary of the penetration of solar energy into Caucasian skin. Less than 10% of UVB (300 nm) is transmitted through the epidermis, compared to nearly 50% of UVA (350 nm) and 50 to 75% of visible light. Only in the far infrared range does transmission begin to decrease with increasing wavelength. Dermal thickness varies from approximately 1 mm (shown in the figure) to approximately 4 mm, depending on body site. Solar elastosis is characteristically most severe at a depth of approximately 0.2 to 0.3 mm. (Modified and reproduced with permission from Parrish, J. A., et al., *UV-A: Biological Effects of Ultraviolet Radiation with Emphasis on Human Responses to Longwave Ultraviolet*, Plenum Press, New York, 1978.)

irradiation period the elastotic dermis was progressively compressed downward by a zone of new collagen and elastin fibers similar to those seen pre-irradiation, suggesting repair.[31]

In an attempt to produce elastosis experimentally in man, previously nonexposed areas of four elderly Caucasians were separately irradiated with predominantly UVC, predominantly UVB, and predominantly UVA after topical application of psoralen (PUVA) on alternate days for 6 to 12 months.[45] Neither routine nor special histochemical stains showed any change beyond epidermal hyperpigmentation. The investigators concluded from this discouraging effort that either much longer induction times were necessary or that older individuals were less capable than children or young adults of responding the repeated UV insults with increased elastin synthesis.

The possibility that clinical changes of "actinic aging" could be reversed by transplanting affected skin to nondamaged sun-protected sites was examined inconclusively in two early studies.[46,47] This question has not been re-explored with contemporary methodologies, probably because current thinking favors direct "primary" sun-induced damage to cells in both the epidermis and dermis, rather than effects in one compartment primarily with secondary effects in the other.

The relationship between chronologic aging and chronic sun damage in the skin has also

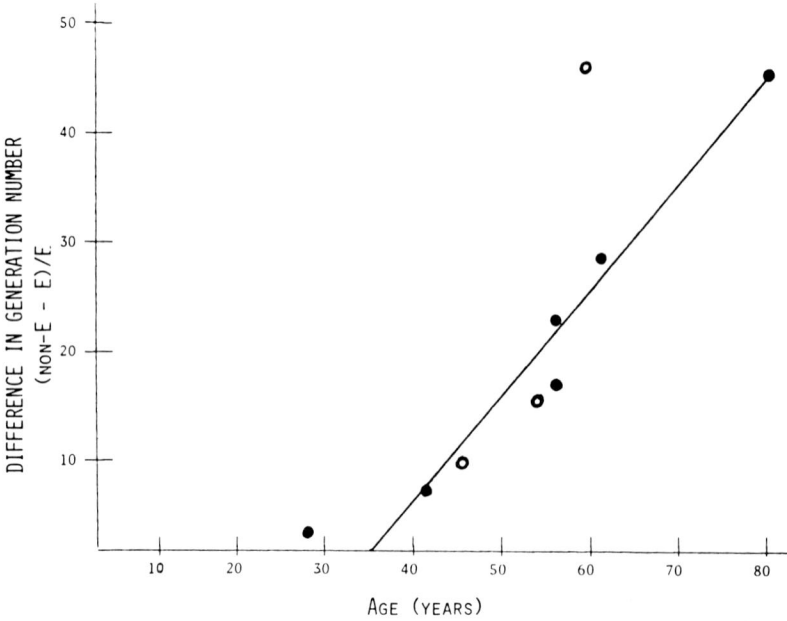

FIGURE 10.   Discrepancy in the average number of generations achieved in culture by keratinocytes from habitually sun-exposed vs. nonexposed skin of the arm (closed circles) and face (open circles). Paired cultures derived from each subject were maintained under identical conditions in vitro and serially passaged until senescence. Older subjects with more severe dermatoheliosis manifest greater differences in generation number between the sun-exposed and nonexposed sites than do younger subjects. The regression line is calculated from the arm-derived cultures only. (Reproduced with permission from Gilchrest, B. A., et al., *J. Invest. Dermatol.*, 80, 81S, 1983.)

been explored in cell culture systems. As discussed in Chapter 7, the in vitro life span and cumulative population doublings (CPD) of human dermal fibroblasts have been found to vary inversely with donor age for healthy adults and to be shortened compared to age-matched controls for individuals with certain "premature aging" syndromes.[48,50-53] Working from the hypothesis that advanced physiologic age is manifested at the cellular level as decreased life span and proliferative capacity in culture, experiments were undertaken to compare cells derived from habitually sun-exposed skin and sun-protected skin of the same individuals. Both keratinocyte[11,54] and fibroblast[55] cultures were established from paired biopsies of the lateral (sun-exposed) and medial (nonexposed) aspects of the upper arm of healthy, well-screened volunteers. In vitro life span, measured as CPD, was in all instances less for cultures derived from the sun-exposed site than for cultures derived from the nonexposed site, and the discrepancy between the two sites increased with age and clinical severity of sun damage (Figures 10 and 11). No subject had been recently sun-exposed. Similar results were obtained with additional sets of keratinocyte cultures derived from paired pre-auricular (sun-exposed) and post-auricular (nonexposed) sites.[28] Hence, in this system habitual sun exposure can indeed be said to accelerate cellular aging by the criterion of decreased culture life span. However, in the case of keratinocytes, for which plating efficiency was also determined, the paired cultures differed in a second way, not interpretable as sun-induced "accelerated aging". In all instances, cultures derived from sun-exposed sites had a higher plating efficiency, i.e., yielded more colonies, than the paired cultures derived from nonexposed sites. Differences were greater for paired cultures derived from the arm of male subjects than from the face of female subjects, but increased with donor

Effect of Donor Age on <u>In Vitro</u> Lifespan of Human Skin Fibroblasts

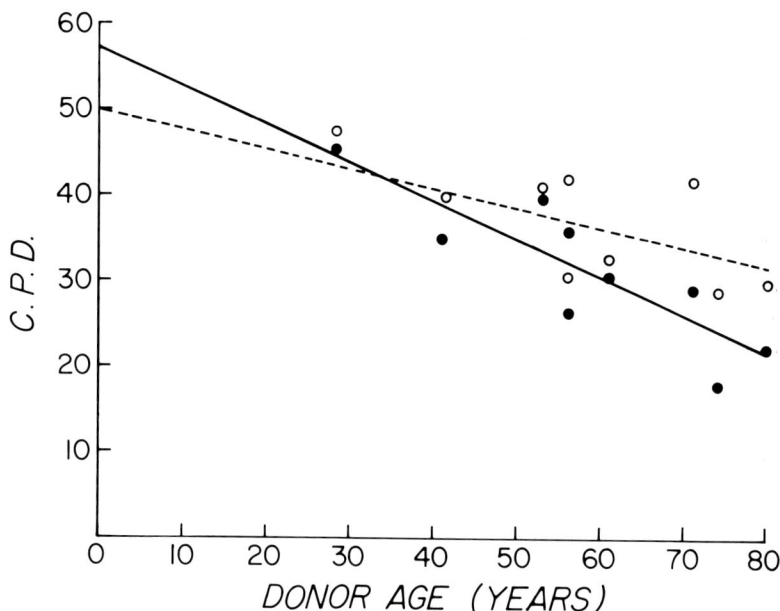

A

FIGURE 11.   Effect of donor age and prior habitual sun exposure on the in vitro life span of dermal fibroblasts. Fibroblast cultures were derived from paired skin biopsies of the lateral (sun-exposed) and medial (nonexposed) aspects of the upper arm of healthy fair-skinned adult subjects and serially passaged under uniform conditions until senescence. Upper panel: (A) Cumulative population doublings (CPD) for paired dermal fibroblast strains plotted as a function of donor age. For each pair, CPD are greater for strains derived from the nonexposed site (open circles) than from the sun-exposed site (closed circles). (B) Discrepancy in culture life span for paired fibroblast strains as a function of donor age. Older subjects with more severe dermatoheliosis have a greater difference in CPD between the two sites than do younger subjects. (Modified by inclusion of additional data and reproduced with permission from Gilchrest, B. A., *J. Gerontol.*, 35, 537, 1980.)

age in both groups[28] (Figure 12). The mechanism of this greater adaptive and/or proliferative behavior by habitually sun-exposed keratinocytes is not known, but may reflect an early step in malignant transformation.[11]

Clinical and histologic changes, apparently an exaggeration of those seen in dermatoheliosis, have been described in workers with long-term occupational tar exposure[56] and in patients receiving methoxalen photochemotherapy (PUVA) for psoriasis.[57-60] Although the two conditions differ slightly from each other, both feature to variable degrees wrinkling, irregular pigmentation, elastosis, and an increased risk of squamous cell carcinoma.[56,61] The existence of UVA-mediated[33] chronic phototoxicity syndromes which closely mimic dermatoheliosis is of theoretic interest and offers the possibility of further insights into the mechanism of sun-induced cutaneous damage.

VI. SIMILARITIES BETWEEN CUTANEOUS AGING AND DERMATOHELIOSIS

The popular confusion between these entities has already been discussed. It must be noted, however, that while the clinical manifestations of aging and chronic sun damage differ, in

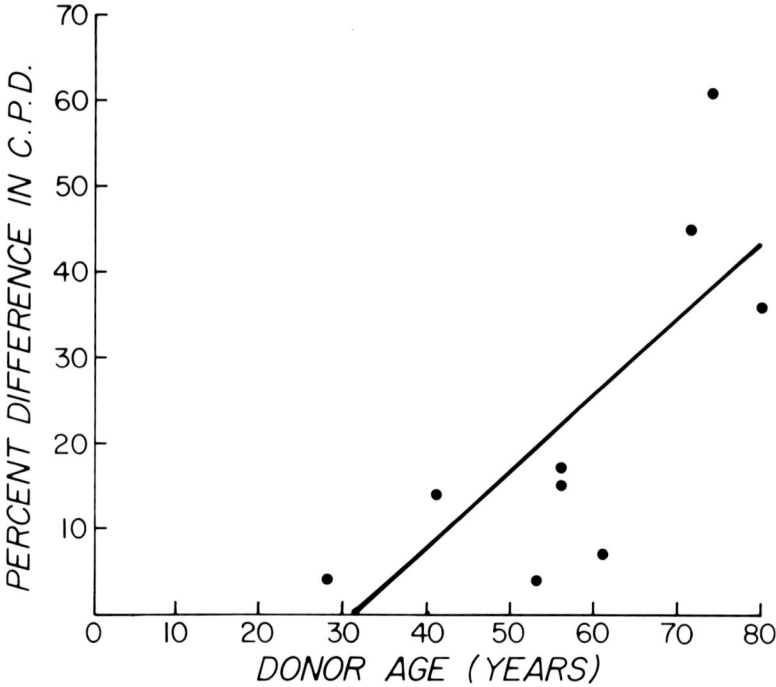

Effect of Chronic Sun Exposure <u>In Vivo</u> on the Lifespan of Cultured Human Fibroblasts

FIGURE 11B

many instances these differences are subtle. Histologically, epidermal and dermal changes in elderly sun-exposed skin have been described by experienced investigators as differing in degree only from those in elderly sun-protected skin, at both the light microscopic and electron microscopic levels.[17,62] Only recently have *qualitative* differences in the dermal fibrous proteins and microvasculature of such paired sites been documented.[18,21] Similarly, cells derived from chronically sun-damaged skin manifest certain in vitro behaviors suggestive of acclerated physiologic aging.[11,55] On a theoretic level, it is interesting to note that several of the mechanisms known to be involved in UV-mediated cellular damage are also postulated to underlie chronologic aging. These include DNA injury and/or decreased DNA repair,[63-65] lysosomal disruption,[66-68] and altered collagen structure.[69-71] These presumed common pathways strengthen the argument often formulated on clinical grounds that chronic sun-exposure truly accelerates aging in the skin and does not merely superimpose unrelated damage on senescent changes.

VII. PREVENTION AND TREATMENT

Avoidance of all sunlight should completely prevent dermatoheliosis, although most individuals do receive appreciable lifetime exposure to portions of the solar spectrum from artificial lighting, various heating sources, and other occupational or recreational encounters. From a realistic viewpoint, complete avoidance of sunlight throughout life would be extremely difficult and unpleasant. However, as discussed in Chapter 6, many practical, effective, and cosmetically elegant sunscreens are currently available either as discrete

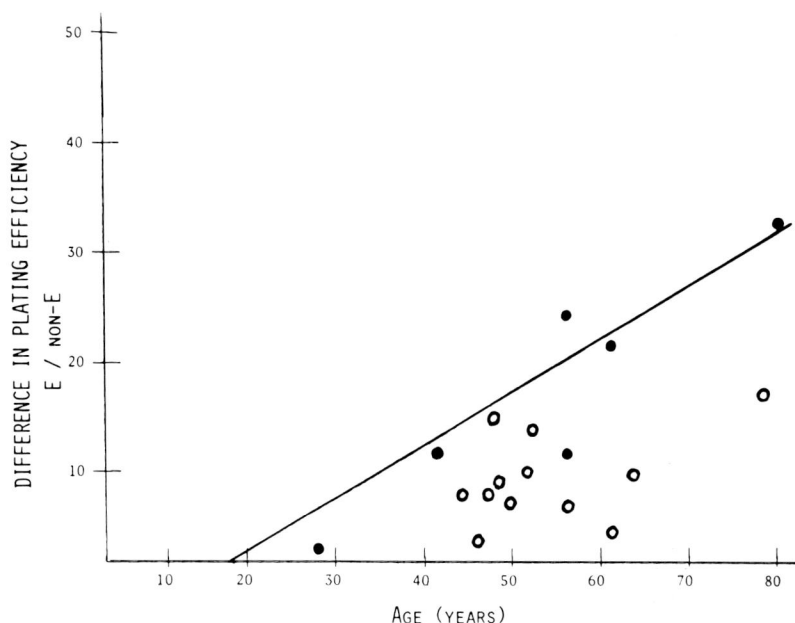

FIGURE 12.   Differences in plating efficienty (P.E.) for primary cultures of keratinocytes from habitually sun-exposed (E) sites on the arm (closed circles) and face (open circles) vs. paired nonexposed (non-E) sites of the same subjects. From each skin specimen, 10^4 disaggregated cells were plated and maintained under standardized conditions, and after 3 weeks the number of colonies was determined: P. E. = no. colonies/10^{-4}. The regression line is calculated from the arm-derived cultures only. Paired cultures derived from pre-auricular (E) and post-auricular (non-E) facelift specimens manifest less difference in P.E., up to 10-fold, than do paired cultures from the lateral (E) and medial (non-E) aspects of the arm, up to 32-fold, but in both sets of cultures there is a progressive increase in the discrepancy with advancing donor age and increasing severity of actinic damage. (Reproduced with permission from Gilchrest, B. A., et al., *J. Invest. Dermatol.,* 80, 81S, 1983.)

products or as components of make-up foundations. Again, in the absence of relevant data, a broad spectrum UV screen would appear more desirable than one directed at either UV-B or UV-A preferentially. Opaque products (including make-up), effective against both UV and visible light, are cosmetically unacceptable to many but not all potential users. Avoidance of excessive infrared irradiation would also seem prudent.

Treatment of dermatoheliosis spans the disciplines of dermatology and plastic surgery. No single approach is appropriate for all its manifestations, and a full discussion of the subject is well beyond the scope of this chapter. Table 2 lists the conventional approaches by component lesions. Anecdotally, cessation of excessive sun-exposure alone allows regression of most epidermal and some dermal lesions even in the absence of therapy. Conversely, there is a strong clinical impression among physicians involved in the treatment of this disorder that ''ablative'' procedures such as dermabrasion or chemical peels may actually exacerbate certain lesions (e.g., telangiectasia and irregular epidermal pigmentation), presumably through further injury to the involved structures.

Table 2
TREATMENT OF DERMATOHELIOSIS

Component lesions	Effective therapies
Dryness (roughness)	Emollients (transient effect)
Actinic keratoses	Topical 5-fluorouracil; cryotherapy; dermabrasion/chemical peel (TCA)
Freckling	Hydroquinone (2-5%)[a]
Lentigenes	Cryotherapy; hydroquinone[a]
Guttate hypomelanosis	NR
Wrinkles	
Fine surface lines	Chemical peel (TCA)
Deep furrows	Rhydidectomy (face lift)
Stellate pseudoscars	NR
Elastosis	NR
Inelasticity (redundant skin)	Rhydidectomy
Telangiectasia	Electrocautery; argon laser
Venous lakes	NR
Purpura	NR
Comedones	Retin-A® (all-trans retinoic acid); manual expression
Sebaceous hyperplasia	Excision

Note: NR = None Reported.

[a] Minimally effective for most patients.

REFERENCES

1. **Lever, W. F.,** Degrenerative disease: senile degeneration, in *Histopathology of the Skin,* 3rd ed., J. B. Lippincott, Philadelphia, 1961, 200.
2. **Kligman, A. M.,** Early destructive effect of sunlight on human skin, *JAMA,* 210, 2377, 1969.
3. **Parrish, J. A., White, H. A. D., and Pathak, M. A.,** Photomedicine: long-term effects of UV radiation, in *Dermatology in General Medicine,* Fitzpatrick, T. B., Eisen, A. Z., Wolff, K., Freedberg, I. M., and Austen, K. F., Eds., McGraw-Hill, New York, 1979, 958.
4. **Nikolsky, P.,** Cutis rhomboidea hypertrophica cervicis, *Z. Haut Geschlechtskr.,* 17, 326, 1925.
5. **Smith, J. G., Jr. and Lansing, A. I.,** Distribution of solar elastosis (senile elastosis) in the skin, *J. Gerontol.,* 14, 496, 1959.
6. **Knox, J. M., Cockerall, E. G., and Freeman, R. B.,** Etiological factors and premature aging, *JAMA,* 179, 630, 1962.
7. **Smith, J. G. and Finlayson, G. R.,** Dermal connective tissue alterations with age and chronic sun damage, *J. Soc. Cosmet. Chem.,* 16, 527, 1965.
8. **Tan, C. Y., Stratham, B., Marks, R., and Payne, P. A.,** Skin thickness measurement by pulsed ultrasound: its reproducibility, validation, and variability, *Br. J. Dermatol.,* 106, 657, 1982.
9. **Pochi, P. E., Strauss, J. S., and Downing, D. T.,** Age-related changes in sebaceous gland activity, *J. Invest. Dermatol.,* 73, 108, 1979.
10. **Lever, W. F.,** *Histopathology of the Skin,* 5th ed., J. B. Lippincott, Philadelphia, 1975.
11. **Gilchrest, B. A.,** Relationship between actinic damage and chronologic aging in keratinocyte cultures of human skin, *J. Invest. Dermatol.,* 72(5), 219, 1979.
12. **Hodgson, C.,** Lentigo senilis, *Arch. Dermatol.,* 87, 197, 1963.
13. **Clark, W. H., Jr. and Mihm, M. C., Jr.,** Lentigo maligna and lentigo-maligna melanoma, *Am. J. Pathol.,* 55, 39, 1969.
14. **McGovern, V. J., Mihm, M. C., Jr., Bailly, C., et al.,** The classification of malignant melanoma and its histologic reporting, *Cancer,* 32, 1446, 1973.

15. **Korting, G. W.,** *Geriatric Dermatology,* translated by Curth, W. and Curth, H. O., W. B. Saunders, Philadelphia, 1980.

16. **Mitchell, R. E.,** Chronic solar dermatosis: a light and electron microscopic study of the dermis, *J. Invest. Dermatol.,* 43, 203, 1967.

16a. **Kligman, A. M.,** Solar elastosis in relation to pigmentation, in *Sunlight and Man,* Pathak, M. A., et al., Eds., University of Tokyo Press, Tokyo, 1974, 157.

17. **Lavker, R. M.,** Structural alterations in exposed and unexposed aged skin, *J. Invest. Dermatol.,* 73, 59, 1979.

18. **Braverman, I. M. and Fonferko, E.,** Studies in cutaneous aging. I. The elastic fiber network, *J. Invest. Dermatol.,* 78, 434, 1982.

19. **Felsher, A.,** Observations on senile elastosis, *J. Invest. Dermatol.,* 37, 163, 1961.

20. **Findlay, G. H.,** On elastase and the elastic dystrophies of the skin, *Br. J. Dermatol.,* 66, 16, 1954.

21. **Braverman, I. M. and Fonferko, E.,** Studies in cutaneous aging. II. The microvasculature, *J. Invest. Dermatol.,* 78, 444, 1982.

22. **Epstein, J. H., Tuffanelli, D. L., and Epstein, W. K.,** Cutaneous changes in the porphyrias, *Arch. Dermatol.,* 107, 689, 1973.

23. **Favre, M. and Racouchot, J.,** L'elasteidose cutanee nodulaire a kystes et a comedones, *Ann. Derm. Syph.,* 78, 681, 1951.

24. **Helm, F.,** Nodular cutaneous elastosis with cysts and comedones (Favre-Racouchot Syndrome), *Arch. Dermatol.,* 84, 666, 1961.

25. **Ramos e Silva, J. and Portugal, H.,** Sur l'adenome sebace senile, *Ann. Derm. Syph.,* 80, 121, 1953.

26. **Gilchrest, B. A., Blog, B. F., and Szabo, G.,** The effect of aging and chronic ultraviolet irradiation on melanocytes in human skin, *J. Invest. Dermatol.,* 75, 1, 1980.

27. **Gilchrest, B. A., Murphy, G., and Soter, N. A.,** Effects of chronologic aging and ultraviolet irradiation on Langerhans cells in human skin, *J. Invest. Dermatol.,* 79, 85, 1982.

28. **Gilchrest, B. A., Szabo, G., Flynn, E., and Goldwyn, R. M.,** Chronologic and actinically induced aging in human facial skin, *J. Invest. Dermatol.,* 80, 81S, 1983.

29. **Delo, V. A., Dawes, L., and Jackson, R.,** Density of Langerhans cells (LC) in normal vs. chronic actinically damaged skin (CADS) in human, *J. Invest. Dermatol.,* 76, 330, 1981.

30. **Sams, W. M., Mitchell, W. S., Jr., Smith, J. G., and Burk, P. G.,** The experimental production of elastosis with ultraviolet light, *J. Invest. Dermatol.,* 43, 467, 1964.

31. **Kligman, L. H., Akin, F. J., and Kligman, A. M.,** Prevention of ultraviolet damage to the dermis of hairless mice by sunscreens, *J. Invest. Dermatol.,* 78, 181, 1982.

32. **Nakamura, K. and Johnson, W. C.,** Ultraviolet light induced connective tissue changes in rat skin: a histopathologic and histochemical study, *J. Invest. Dermatol.,* 51(4), 253, 1968.

33. **Parrish, J. A., Anderson, R. R., Urback, F., and Pitts, D.,** UV-A: *Biological Effects of Ultraviolet Radiation with Emphasis on Human Responses to Longwave Ultraviolet,* Plenum Press, New York, 1978.

34. **Bener, P.,** Spectral intensity of natural ultraviolet radiation and its dependence on various parameters, in *The Biologic Effects of Ultraviolet Radiation,* Urbach, F., Ed., Plenum Press, New York, 1969, 351.

35. **Gates, D. M.,** Spectral distribution of solar radiation at the earth's surface, *Science,* 151, 523, 1966.

36. **Blum, H. F.,** *Carcinogenesis by Ultraviolet Light,* Princeton University Press, Princeton, 1959.

37. **Sayre, R. M., Olson, R. L., and Everett, M. A.,** Quantitative studies on erythema, *J. Invest. Dermatol.,* 46, 240, 1966.

38. **Smith, J. G., Jr., Davidson, E. A., Tindall, J. G., and Sams, W. M., Jr.,** Hexosamine and hydroxyproline alterations in chronically sun-damaged skin, *Proc. Soc. Exp. Biol. Med.,* 108, 533, 1961.

39. **Sorbel, H., Gabay, S., Wright, E. T., Lichtenstein, I., and Nelson, N. H.,** The influence of age upon the hexosamine collagen ratio of dermal biopsies, *J. Gerontol.,* 13, 128, 1958.

40. **Smith, J. G., Jr., Davidson, E. A., and Clark, R. D.,** Dermal elastin in actinic elastosis and pseudoxanthoma elasticum, *Nature (London),* 195, 716, 1962.

41. **Felsher, A.,** Observations on senile elastosis, *J. Invest. Dermatol.,* 37, 163, 1961.

42. **Smith, J. G., Jr., Davidson, E. A., Sams, W. M., Jr., and Clark, R. D.,** Alterations in human dermal connective tissue with age and chronic sun damage, *J. Invest. Dermatol.,* 39, 342, 1962.

43. **Hargis, A. M., Thomassen, R. W., and Phemister, R. D.,** Chronic dermatosis and cutaneous squamous cell carcinoma in the beagle dog, *Vet. Pathol.,* 14, 218, 1977.

44. **Berger, H., Tsamboas, D., and Mahrel, G.,** Experimental elastosis induced by chronic ultraviolet exposure, *Arch. Dermatol. Res.,* 269, 39, 1980.

45. **Shellow, W. V. R. and Kligman, A. M.,** An attempt to produce elastosis in aged human skin by means of ultraviolet irradiation, *J. Invest. Dermatol.,* 50, 225, 1968.

46. **Gerstein, W. and Freeman, R. C.,** Transplantation of actinically damaged skin, *J. Invest. Dermatol.,* 41, 445, 1963.

47. **Papa, C. M., Carter, D. M., and Kligman, A. M.,** The effect of autotransplantation on the progression of reversibility of aging in human skin, *J. Invest. Dermatol.,* 54, 200, 1970.
48. **Martin, G. M., Sprague, C. A., and Epstein, C. J.,** Replicative lifespan of cultivated human cells, effects of donor's age, tissue, and genotype, *Lab. Invest.,* 23, 86, 1970.
49. **Schneider, E. L. and Mitsui, Y.,** The relationship between in vitro cellular aging and in vivo human age, *Proc. Natl. Acad. Sci. USA,* 73, 3584, 1976.
50. **Goldstein, S.,** Lifespan of cultured cells in progeria, *Lancet,* 1, 424, 1969.
51. **Danes, B. S.,** Progeria: a cell culture study on aging, *J. Clin. Invest.,* 50, 2000, 1971.
52. **Goldstein, S., Littlefield, J. W., and Woeldner, J. S.,** Diabetes mellitus and aging: diminished plating efficiency of cultured human fibroblasts, *Proc. Natl. Acad. Sci. USA,* 64, 155, 1969.
53. **Goldstein, S. and Moerman, E. J.,** Chronologic and physiologic age affect replicative life-span of fibroblasts from diabetic, prediabetic and normal donors, *Science,* 781, 1977.
54. **Gilchrest, B. A.,** A quantitative approach to measuring actinic aging in human skin, *J. Soc. Cosmet. Chem.,* 32, 153, 1981.
55. **Gilchrest, B. A.,** Prior chronic sun exposure decreases the lifespan of human skin fibroblasts in vitro, *J. Gerontol.,* 35, 537, 1980.
56. **Geitz, H.,** Tar keratosis, in *Cancer of the Skin,* Andrade, R., Gumport, S. L., Papkin, G. L., and Rees, T. D., Eds., W. B. Saunders, Philadelphia, 1976, 437.
57. **Bergfeld, W.,** Histopathologic changes in the skin after photochemotherapy, *Cutis,* 20, 504, 1977.
58. **Hashimoto, K., Kohda, H., Kumakira, M., Blender, S., and Willis, I.,** Psoralen-UVA-treated psoriatic lesions, *Arch. Dermatol.,* 114, 711, 1978.
59. **Gschnait, F., Wolff, K., Honigsmann, H., Stingl, G., Brenner, W., Jaschke, E., and Konrad, K.,** Long-term photochemotherapy: histopathological and immunofluorescence observations in 243 patients, *Br. J. Dermatol.,* 103, 11, 1980.
60. **Zelickson, A. S., Mottaz, J. H., Zelickson, B. D., and Muller, S. A.,** Elastic tissue changes in skin following PUVA therapy, *J. Am. Acad. Dermatol.,* 3, 186, 1980.
61. **Stern, R. S., Thibodeau, L. A., Kleinerman, R. A., Parrish, J. A., and Fitzpatrick, T. B.,** Risk of cutaneous carcinoma in patients treated with oral methoxsalen photochemotherapy for psoriasis, *N. Engl. J. Med.,* 300, 809, 1979.
62. **Montagna, W. and Carlisle, K.,** Structural changes in aging human skin, *J. Invest. Dermatol.,* 73, 47, 1979.
63. **Cleaver, J. E.,** DNA damage and repair in light sensitive human skin disease, *J. Invest. Dermatol.,* 54, 181, 1970.
64. **Hart, R. W. and Setlow, R. B.,** Correlation between deoxyribonucleic acid excision-repair and lifespan in a number of mammalian species, *Proc. Natl. Acad. Sci. USA,* 71, 2169, 1974.
65. **Cutler, R. G.,** Crosslinkage hypothesis of aging: DNA adducts in chromatin as a primary aging process, in *Aging, Carcinogenesis and Radiation Biology,* Smith, K. C., Ed., Plenum Press, New York, 1975, 443.
66. **Johnson, B. E. and Daniels, F., Jr.,** Lysosomes and the action of skin to ultraviolet light, *J. Invest. Dermatol.,* 53, 85, 1969.
67. **Daniels, F., Jr. and Johnson, B. E.,** Normal, physiologic, and pathologic effects of solar radiation on the skin, in *Sunlight and Man,* Fitzpatrick, T. B., et al., Eds., University of Tokyo Press, Tokyo, 1974, 117.
68. **Cristafalo, V. J., Howard, B. V., and Kritschevsky, D.,** *Inorganic Biological and Medicinal Chemistry,* Gallo, X. and Santamaria, L., Eds., North-Holland, Amsterdam, 1970, 95.
69. **Bottoms, E. and Shuster, S.,** Effect of ultraviolet light on skin collagen, *Nature (London),* 199, 192, 1963.
70. **Sams, W. M., Jr. and Smith, J. G., Jr.,** Alterations in human dermal fibrous connective tissue with age and chronic sun damage, in *Advances in Biology of the Skin,* Vol. 6, Aging, Montagna, W., Ed., Pergamon Press, Oxford, 1965, 199.
71. **Bjorkstein, J.,** The crosslinkage theory of aging, *Finska Kensists Medd.,* 80, 23, 1971.
72. **Kligman, A. M.,** personal communication.

INDEX